THE COMPLETE PHOTO GUIDE TO
SOAP MAKING

This book is dedicated to soap makers past and present—from the mythical washerwomen of Mount Sapo, to the chandlers of the Middle Ages, to the pioneers of the 1970s, to the hundreds of thousands of soap makers today. We have all been enchanted by this seemingly common, yet endlessly inspiring, substance.

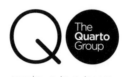

Inspiring | Educating | Creating | Entertaining

Brimming with creative inspiration, how-to projects, and useful information to enrich your everyday life, quarto.com is a favorite destination for those pursuing their interests and passions.

First published in 2018 by Creative Publishing international, an imprint of The Quarto Group, 100 Cummings Center, Suite 265-D, Beverly, MA 01915, USA.
T (978) 282-9590 F (978) 283-2742 Quarto.com

10 9 8 7 6 5 4

ISBN: 978-1-58923-943-2

Digital edition published in 2018.
Library of Congress Cataloging-in-Publication Data available.
Design and Page Layout: Laura McFadden Design, Inc.
Photography: Glenn Scott Photography, except for project step-shots by David Fisher Packaging shown on page 139 (clockwise from top left): Sarah Nesbitt, Irene Linauer, and Charlene Simon.

Printed in China

For your safety, use caution, care, and good judgment when following the procedures described in this book. The publisher and author cannot assume responsibility for any damage to property or injury to persons as a result of misuse of the information provided.

THE COMPLETE PHOTO GUIDE TO
SOAP MAKING

DAVID FISHER

Creative Publishing international

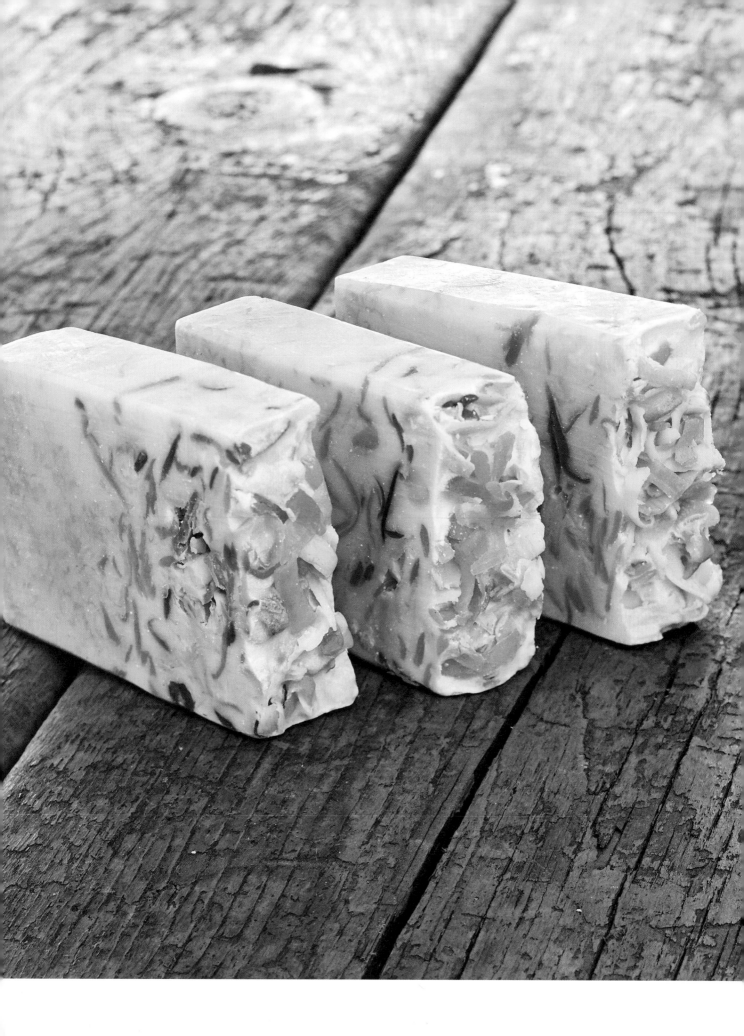

Contents

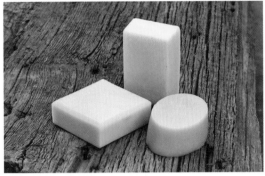

Introduction

I have always been a crafty person. As a child, I built models, did macramé, and carved wood. As an adult, it was no surprise, then, when a craft-themed book club advertisement came in the mail, that I joined. One book I chose was on making soap, and, practically from the first pages, I was hooked. To me, soap making is this amazing blend of science, art, frugal living, craftmaking, cooking, creativity, health, emotion, and more—all combined into a product you use every day. It can be practical and functional as well as sensual and exciting, and every day when you hold it in your hand, you can say, "I made that." Then it will wash down the drain and you will have to make some more.

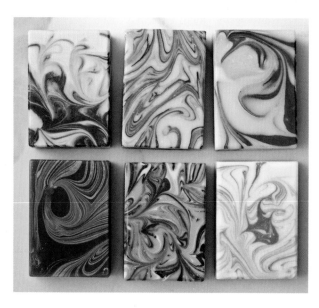

This book covers all the major concepts and types of soap making. The projects and recipes come from years of time in the kitchen and sharing with other soap makers. But the most important thing about the techniques and information contained here is that you take them and make them your own. Start with the basics, but don't stay there. A world of inspiring ingredients, colors, scents, additives, and shapes awaits.

You are about to enter a world of more delightful and luxurious baths and showers—a hobby (or business) that will inspire you for many years. You are joining a community of fellow soap-making "addicts" who love the craft as much as you will. You will look at the world through new glasses—seeing random containers as possible molds; seeing colors or patterns in food or art and wondering how you can duplicate them in soap. Every spice in your cabinet, vegetable in your garden, and beverage in your refrigerator will be looked at differently: Can I add it (and what would it do) to a batch? Your kitchen will be messy, but your heart will be full, and your friends will secretly wonder when you are going to bring them more.

A Brief History of Soap and Soap Making

A popular soap-making legend attributes the origins of soap to Mount Sapo in Rome, where animal sacrifices would take place and the melted animal fat would mix with the wood ashes. This crude "soap" would then wash down the hill into the river below where the servant women discovered that it helped clean their garments better. Alas, it doesn't appear there ever was a Mount Sapo, but the gist of the story is true—people discovering that water, ashes, and oil combine to make a substance that makes washing things easier.

Evidence of soap and soap-like materials has been found in ancient Babylon, Egypt, and Rome. (*Sapo* is Latin for soap.) In medieval times, there are references to the trade and manufacture of soap in the Middle East and Europe. From the fifteenth through eighteenth centuries, the production of soap increased in both factory production and through guilds of chandlers who would collect tallow and fat from butchers, or door to door, and make soap and candles from them.

The nineteenth century brought breakthroughs for the soap-making industry with the development of commercially made lye—no more need for wood ashes—and the industrial revolution. Soap companies, such as Pears, Lever Brothers, B.J. Johnson, and others made soap a common, affordable household item.

The next breakthrough (or setback) for soap came because of the World Wars. Fats, like most supplies, were in short supply, especially because glycerin could be extracted from them to make nitroglycerin explosives. Synthetic detergents were developed to fill the gap and, throughout the 1950s, '60s, and '70s, became commonplace, both as household and personal cleansers.

Most soap makers mark the beginning of the modern handcrafted soap making renaissance with the publication of a small book in 1972 by Ann Bramson, simply titled *Soap*. Since then, the art, craft, hobby, and business of soap making has grown considerably, and people around the world are finding the same joy that those mythical washerwomen of Mount Sapo must have experienced when they discovered the delight of handmade soap.

Basic Soap-Making Methods and Types of Soap

Soap making certainly has come a long way since the days of boiling grease and ashes in giant pots outdoors. But the basic chemical equation is the same:

Soaps Using a Premade Base

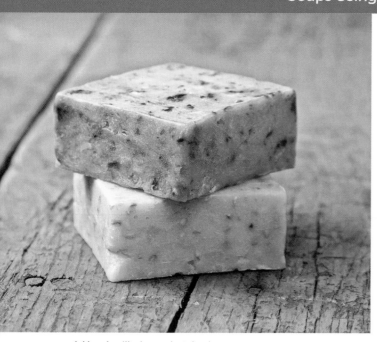

1. Hand-milled, or rebatched, soap

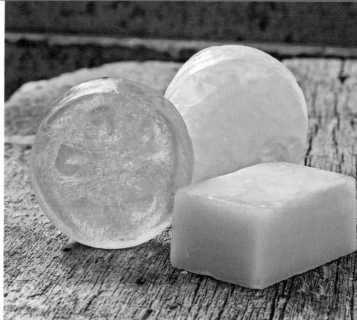

2. Melt-and-pour soap

Hand-Milled, or Rebatched, Soap

Hand-milled soap (sometimes called rebatched soap) starts with a grated or chopped premade batch of either cold process or hot process soap that is slowly heated until it liquefies into a moldable mixture. It's a good method for making just a couple of bars to test a fragrance or colorant, as well as to rescue a problem batch of soap. It's like melt-and-pour soap (following) in that you start with already made soap and customize it with your own scents, colors, and additives.

Melt-and-Pour Soap

Melt-and-pour soap also uses a real soap base (made with oils and lye), but includes additional ingredients in the soap that allow it to melt when heated. As with hand-milled soap, you don't have to measure or mix the oils yourself, you just melt the premade base, add the colors, fragrances, and additives you want, and pour it into a mold. Think of it like a plain cake mix that you customize into your own unique creation.

The other benefits of melt-and-pour soap are the widespread availability of transparent bases, as well as how easily they liquefy, which allow for soap designs not possible with other methods.

oils (or fats) + lye (and some water) = soap (along with some glycerin—a humectant that's a natural by-product of the soap-making process).

There are four basic methods you can use to make soap: two use premade soap as a starting point and two make soap from scratch.

Soaps Made from Scratch

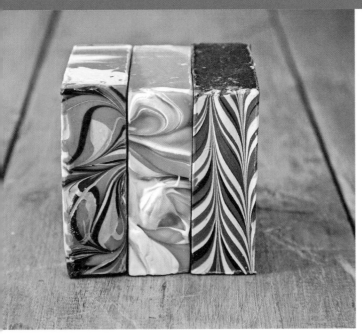

3. Cold process soap

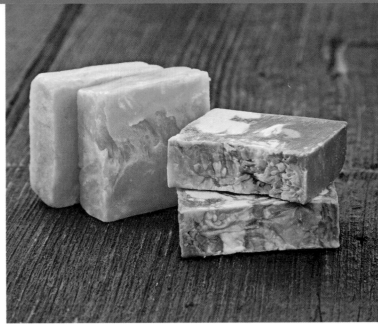

4. Hot process soap

Cold Process Soap

Cold process is, perhaps, the most common method for making soap from scratch. Starting with melted oils and a lye solution, the soap is mixed, and additives, such as scent and color, are added. The soap is placed in a mold and set aside while *saponification*—the chemical reaction that turns the soap mixture into a solid—takes place. This method is called "cold process" because no additional heat is added after the oils are melted.

Hot Process Soap

The only difference between cold process and hot process soap is the addition of heat *after* the oils and lye are mixed to speed the chemical reaction. Instead of letting the lye and oils combine at their own pace (which generates some heat), heat is added and the chemical reaction is sped up considerably. The heat can be added with a slow cooker, oven, or in a large pot. What we think of as "pioneer" soap making—in a huge black pot over a wood fire—is actually a form of hot process soap making.

Soap-Making Essentials

You don't need a lot of fancy or expensive equipment to start making soap. Most of what you'll need is probably already in your kitchen.

Of course, in addition to some basic ingredients—whether you're using a premade base or raw ingredients to make soap from scratch—you'll need items to measure and stir your ingredients, something to heat them in, any additives you want to include, and, finally, something to mold your soap in.

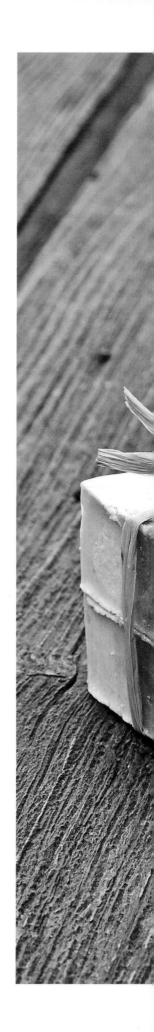

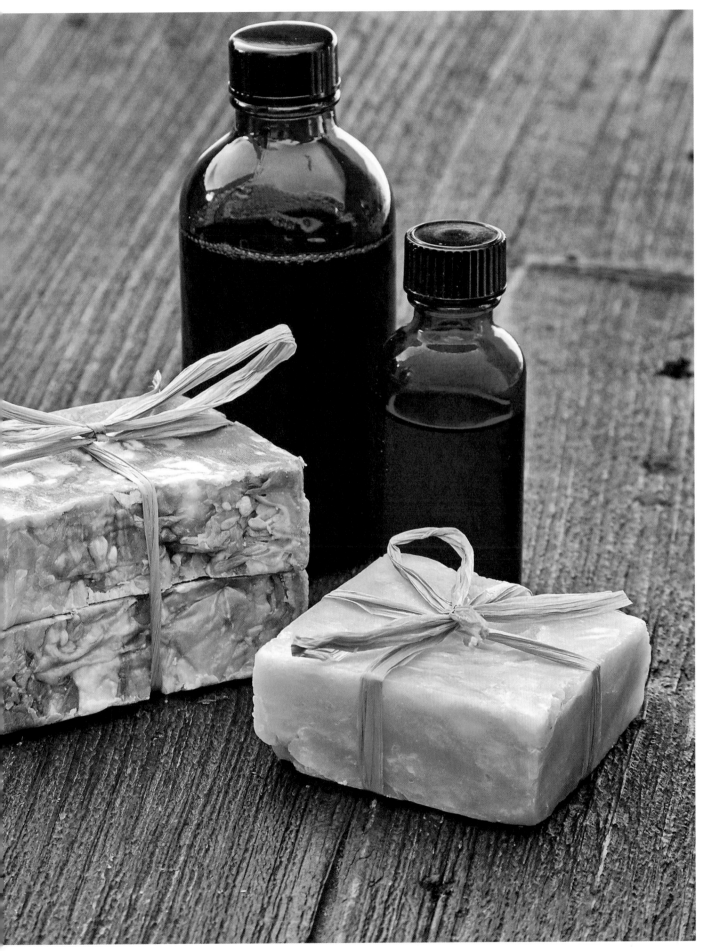

Quick Start Guide: Soap Making Basics

Making soap can be as simple or as complex as you want it to be. You can make simple recipes or delve into the chemistry and details of every fatty acid. If you want to jump right in, here are several important concepts to know.

1   Without lye, there is no soap. Though there should never be any lye left in your soap, lye is required to make the soap in the first place—even melt-and-pour soap is made with lye.

2   Water is a matchmaker. Water allows the lye and oil molecules to combine more easily.

3   The oils in your recipe are the primary determinant of the qualities of your final soap.

4   Weigh everything you reasonably can. Although you will often see tiny amounts of ingredients measured in teaspoons or tablespoons, it's best to weigh as many of your ingredients as possible, *even the liquids*.

5   Natural is not always safe. Just because an ingredient comes directly from nature does not mean it is safe to add to your soap. Conversely, just because something is synthetic does not it mean it is harmful. Know your ingredients.

6   Trace—that "point of no return"—is not as important as it used to be. When soap was mixed by hand, trace was an important point to reach. Trace really could be called *emulsification*, where the lye and oils are fully mixed and won't separate.

7   Be safe, always. Seriously. Lye in your eye is a trip to the emergency room. Don't risk it.

8   When making soap from scratch, always run your recipes through an online lye calculator, such as www.soapcalc.net—even recipes you find in books or online. Errors happen. Typos happen. Plus, you'll learn more about the recipe by double-checking it.

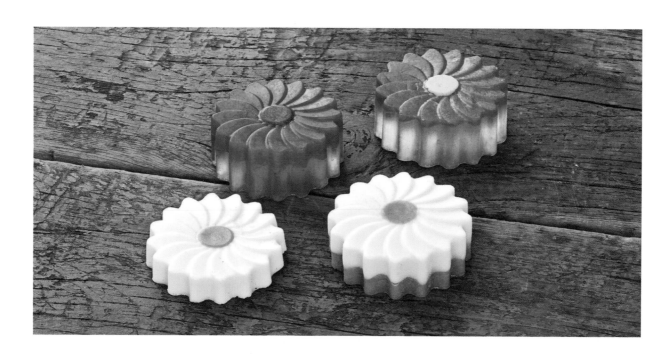

Tempest in a Soap Pot: A Soap-Making Fable

Once upon a time, there was a magical secluded lagoon (also known as your soap pot), cut off from the rest of the ocean, except by one tiny entrance (your measuring cup). The water was pure and clear and just the right temperature (generally about 100°F or 38°C). One day, when the tide was particularly high, 100 oily fish swam through the entrance into the lagoon—35 tuna (olive oil), 30 salmon (coconut oil), 30 mackerel (palm oil), and 5 herring (castor oil). They swam around in the lagoon happily until, one day, 25 hungry caustic sharks (lye) were poured into the lagoon.

The sharks, as you would expect, began devouring the fish. However, every time a shark ate 4 fish, something magical happened. It stopped, shuddered, heated up, and transformed into 4 sturdy, smart dolphins (soap) and a gentle sea turtle (glycerin). The dolphins were all slightly different, depending on the fish that the shark had eaten. This is just like how different oils give soap different qualities. The sharks kept eating the fish until there was nothing left but dolphins and sea turtles. Twenty-five sharks and 100 fish transformed into 100 dolphins and 25 sea turtles. That's the saponification process.

Of course, there are variations to the story.

Once, there were only 96 fish in the lagoon. Twenty-four sharks transformed, but there was still one caustic shark swimming around. This is the same as having too much lye in your soap—it will bite you.

Another time, there were 110 oily fish and the same number of sharks. All the sharks transformed into dolphins and sea turtles, and there were 10 fish left over. This is superfatting—adding more oils (or fish) to the pot than there are sharks (or lye) to consume. Now, a few extra fish are great, but too many (too high a superfat percentage) makes the lagoon crowded and the dolphins very unhappy. So, make sure the lagoon has just enough fish for all the sharks to transform—with just a few left over.

The moral of our soapy lagoon is to keep track of your sharks and fish, and plan for the varieties of dolphins you want swimming around.

Basic Soap-Making Equipment

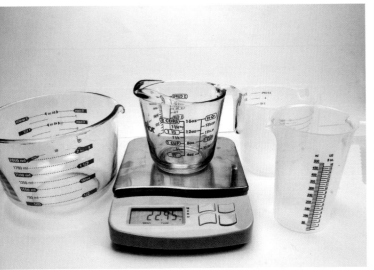
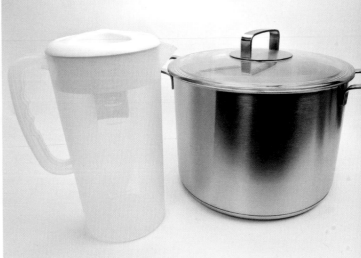

Regardless of which soap-making method you start with, you're going to need the following tools for your basic setup.

First, there are two important rules for all soap making equipment:

1   If you're making soap from scratch with lye, do *not* use any type of metal equipment—containers, bowls, spoons, and so forth—

except those made from stainless steel. Alternatives to stainless steel are high-strength glass (such as Pyrex) or heavy-duty plastic.

2   Do *not* use plastic equipment with undiluted fragrance oil or essential oil. These ingredients can eat right through some plastics. Also, if you use plastic pots, pitchers, or bowls, make sure they can withstand temperatures up to 200°F (93°C).

Preparing for Your First Batch

With any soap-making method, it's recommended that you wear gloves and eye protection. *For cold and hot process, they're required!* For more information, see Making Soap Safely (page 17). No matter how careful you are, wear clothes you don't mind getting a color or oil stain on.

Weighing and Measuring

You'll need a basic kitchen scale to measure ingredients. In soap making, you weigh as many ingredients as you reasonably can, including the liquids. To start with, any scale that measures down to grams or ounces is fine.

Measuring cups are used to separate portions of a soap batch.

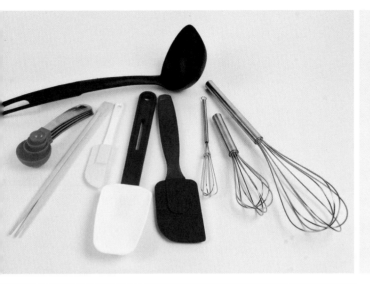

Can I Use the Same Equipment to Make Food and Soap?

In most cases, yes. *Except for the ramekins used to measure fragrances and the pitchers used to make lye solutions*, you don't need to keep two sets of equipment to make food and soap. If you wash everything thoroughly after making soap, it will be fine to use for food.

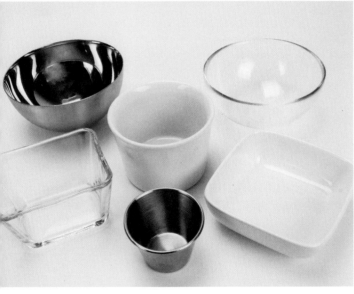

Pots and Pitchers

The size of the soap batches you make will determine which pitchers or pots you'll need. For just a couple of bars, a 2-cup (475 ml) measuring cup is great. For batches that are 2 to 4 pounds (908 g to 1.8 kg), a large measuring pitcher will work. For batches larger than that, you'll need a stainless steel pot.

Spoons, Spatulas, and Whisks

These are used to stir the soap mixture, to mix in colors and fragrances, and to get those last bits of soap out of your pots or pitchers.

Small Bowls and Ramekins

Small bowls or ramekins are useful for mixing colorants or weighing fragrances. Medium-size bowls and measuring cups can be used to separate and color portions of your soap batch.

Paper Towels

Soap making is messy. Always keep several rolls of paper towels on hand for spills, splatters, or any other cleanup you may need to do.

Setting Up a Soap-Making Workspace

There are several key things to do when setting up your soap-making area.

1 Keep it organized. Leaving out an ingredient or spilling one can ruin a batch of soap, as can being unable able to find a particular utensil. Keep all your ingredients, tools, and equipment organized and check to make sure you have everything you need before you start.

2 Keep it clean. Closely related to keeping things organized, all your hard work can be ruined by a stray crumb, pet hair, or piece of random dirt getting into your soap.

3 Keep things protected. In addition to keeping yourself protected, protect your area. Soap-making ingredients can stain, mar, or even eat right through certain materials in your kitchen.

4 Plan ahead and work methodically. Visualize the steps of the whole batch coming together, even going so far as to talk yourself through it. "First I'll mix the oils, then I'll mix in the fragrance oil and the poppy seeds, then I'll separate the batch into these three containers and stir in the color, then I'll pour the lavender first, then the yellow, then the green."

5 A common tip when measuring ingredients is to move them to a different counter, or at least a different place on the counter, after being used. This helps you not forget anything.

Methods to Heat, Melt, and Cook the Ingredients

You'll find most of the equipment needed to make soap in your kitchen. However, there are heating or cooking methods that work better with different methods of soap making.

	MELT AND POUR	COLD PROCESS	HOT PROCESS	HAND MILLED
Microwave Oven	Preferred	Good to heat oils	Only to heat oils	Scorches soap
Pot on Stovetop	Will work, but easy to scorch soap	Good to heat oils	Only to heat oils	Good if using oven-roasting bag
Slow Cooker	Will work, but easy to scorch soap	Slow, but good for keeping oils warm over a longer period of time	Good for cooking soap	Good for reconstituting soap
Pot in Oven	Will work, but not preferred	Slow, but good for keeping oils warm over a longer period of time	Good for cooking soap	Good for reconstituting soap
Double Boiler	Works fine	Not useful	Will work, but not ideal	Good if using oven-roasting bag

Good Manufacturing Practices

As your soap making grows, your best friend will become a notebook of your batches. Write down or print out your recipes and keep them in a binder, noting what and how much of each additive, fragrance, or blend you used, and if there were irregularities. That way, if it comes out fabulously and you want to make that batch again, you'll know exactly what you did. Likewise, if there's a problem, you'll be able to diagnose it more easily.

Even if you think you may never sell your soap, it's a good idea to create a system that documents your batches and your entire process. Think about the process from beginning to end, from ordering the raw ingredients to using the soap, and keep at least basic records of the process. For example:

- Keep all invoices for ingredients.
- Write order dates on all your bottles and tubs of ingredients so you can reference them back to the order.
- Date all your soap recipes and note when you open a new ingredient. This allows you to trace the ingredients in a certain batch back to their source.
- If you have a standard procedure for your process (e.g., temperature to mix), note any variances from it. If you vary things from batch to batch, note all the details of the batch.
- Note the results of the final product. For example:
   o Did you get any ash (see page 143)?
   o Did the colors stay true?
   o Did the colors work well together?
   o Was the scent strong enough?
   o How soon was it hard enough to unmold and cut?

Making Soap Safely

While melt-and-pour and hand-milled soap making may be safer, overall, because you do not deal directly with lye solutions, all methods of soap making have safety concerns. Soap can be made completely safely if you follow these simple rules.

1 Know your ingredients and treat them with respect.

2 Protect yourself and your work area.

3 Educate others in the household about your process and ingredients.

4 Eliminate distractions—pets, children, phone calls, spouses, etc.

5 Prepare for spills—you can never have too many paper towels on hand.

6 Understand the process and the steps before you start.

7 Relax, but stay focused.

Burns

In all soap-making methods, you will deal with hot and heated ingredients. Use proper gloves, hot pads, and trivets so you can work safely with them.

Ingredients

All ingredients in soap making can be worked with safely, but many can cause harm if handled improperly. Lye is considered the most dangerous ingredient in making soap, but one that often gets overlooked is sensitization. Though fragrance and essential oils are safe in a finished bar of soap, when making the soap, these oils are in a very concentrated form. Repeated contact with scents can cause sensitization—essentially developing an allergy to the oil. Always wear gloves when measuring fragrance or essential oils and wipe up any spills carefully. Similarly, be careful of breathing fumes, dust, colorants, or other powders. Though one time may not be an issue, repeated contact may cause problems.

Additives for Soap: Exfoliants

Many natural ingredients can be added to soap as exfoliants to scrub away dead skin cells. As with colorants, the more you add, the more of an effect it creates, both visually and in its scrubbiness. Start with 1 to 2 teaspoons per 1 pound (454 g) of oils or soap base and vary the amount from there based on your preference.

One note of caution: Remember that whatever you put in your soap will end up in the bottom of the shower or bath. Some exfoliants, such as poppy seeds, look great in the bar of soap, but can make a mess in the shower.

- **Calendula petals:** give a light scrub and retain their yellow color nicely.
- **Chamomile flowers:** provide a medium scrub, especially if not finely ground.
- **Citrus peel (dried and ground):** offers a medium scrub; add at trace.
- **Coffee grounds:** scrubbiness is determined by the coffee's grind; brew the grounds first or they will bleed into the soap.
- **Cornmeal:** medium scrub; premix with oil and add at trace.
- **Eucalyptus leaves:** gives a medium scrub, especially if not very finely ground.
- **Lavender buds:** can be used whole for a medium scrub, but will turn brown in cold process soap and look like mouse droppings; gently grind them first to avoid this.
- **Loofah:** light to medium scrub, and can be either whole in a long, round loaf of soap, sliced in an individual bar, or ground and mixed into the soap.
- **Mint:** light scrub, but prone to bleeding; steep as a tea first.
- **Oatmeal:** like coffee, the scrubbiness is determined by how ground it is.
- **Poppy seeds:** light to medium scrub; they look great in the bar of soap, but end up scattered all over the shower or bath.
- **Pumice:** heavy-duty scrub; great for mechanic's or gardener's hand soaps.

- **Rose hips:** medium to high scrub; also adds natural color.
- **Rose petals:** a lovely light to medium scrub, but they turn black in cold process soap.
- **Sandalwood powder:** gives a medium to high scrub, and makes a lovely purple color.
- **Seeds:** ground stone fruit pits (apricots, peaches) and berry seeds (ground or whole) give a medium to high scrub factor.
- **Tea leaves:** provide a light scrub; prone to bleeding so use already steeped leaves.
- **Walnut shells:** ground shells give a nice medium scrub and a lovely medium brown color.

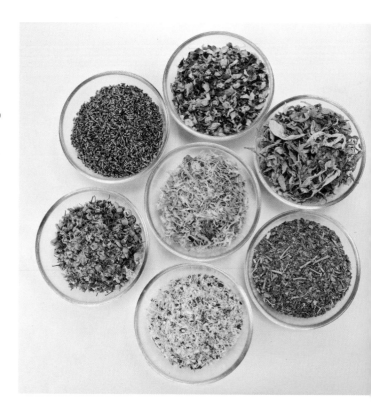

Colorants

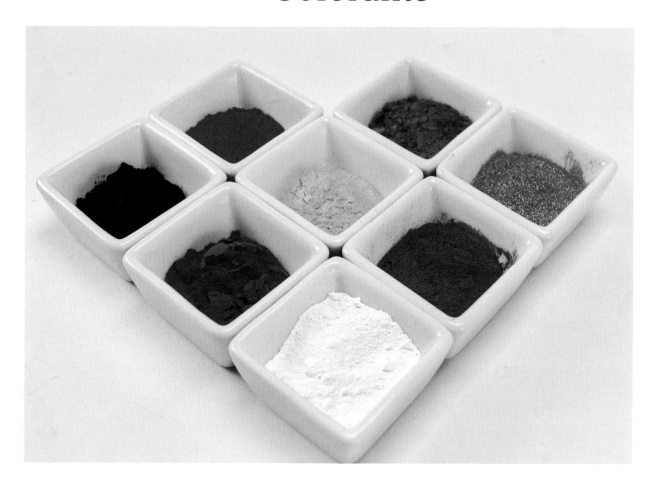

Plain white soap works just as well as brightly colored and swirled soap—the difference is purely visual appeal. But color and design elements transform your soaps from practical to useable works of art.

There are several types of colorants that can be added to soap:

- **Dyes:** Often in liquid form, these colorants give a full range of hues—from subtle to bright and bold. Because they are water soluble, though, they can bleed between layers or swirls of soap, especially in melt-and-pour soap. Some are not stable in cold process soap, so test them first.

- **Oxides and pigments:** Today, these iron-based colorants are synthetic versions instead of being mined from the earth. They have a more "earthy" range of colors, but are very stable and strong in soap.

- **Micas:** It is unclear whether the word "mica" comes from the Latin word *mica,* meaning crumb or grain, or from *micare,* which means "to glitter," but it is a very popular sparkling colorant used in both soap and cosmetics. Micas have a layered crystalline structure and are coated with other oxides, pigments, or dyes to give an even more complex effect.

Scents

Think of a time when you were very happy. Visualize it for a moment.

Chances are, in addition to visualizing it, you also recall what it smelled like. Our sense of smell is connected directly to the forebrain and the limbic system (our primitive lizard brain) and is strongly linked to memories and emotions. Scents can help us feel relaxed, uplifted, energized, and more. Part of their effect is chemical (from which the whole field of aromatherapy stems), and part is mental, through their connections with our emotions.

As soap makers, either in the form of fragrance oils or essential oils, scent is one of the most important and enjoyable additives to our soap.

Essential Oils

Essential oils are just that, the "essence" of a plant. Whether it's the scent from a freshly peeled orange, a crushed sprig of rosemary, or a rose petal, it's the essential oil in them responsible for the scent. It can take hundreds, or even thousands, of pounds of plant material to extract a pound of essential oil. They are used in perfumes, food, cosmetics, household items, and, yes, soap.

Fragrance Oils

Fragrance oils are formulated from a mix of various chemicals. Some of these constituents are natural, coming from plants or animals, and some are

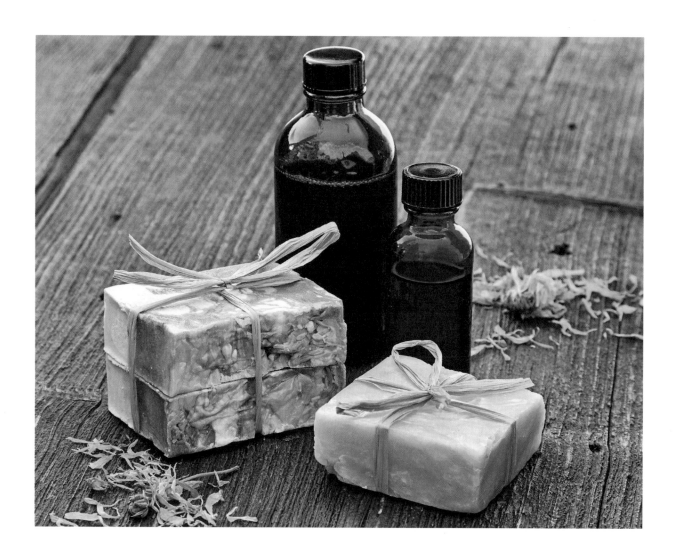

synthetic. Sometimes they are created to smell *like* something occurring in nature (lavender, strawberry shortcake, fresh-cut grass), or sometimes they are created to smell like a feeling or a concept (energy, desert sun, winter moonlight.) Some fragrance oils contain essential oils as part of their makeup and some do not.

Scent Safety

Be sure the fragrance oils or essential oils you use in your soaps are safe to use on your skin. Just because an essential oil is natural, doesn't mean it's safe on your skin. Likewise, just because a fragrance oil is synthetic, doesn't mean it's unsafe.

Using Fragrance Oils and Essential Oils in Soap

As a rule, use the following as a starting place for adding fragrance to your soaps and go from there. Some lighter scents, such as a delicate floral, might need a bit more. Some strong scents, such as peppermint, might need less.

For cold and hot process soaps, start with 0.5 to 0.7 ounce (14 to 20 g) of scent for each pound (454 g) of oils in your recipe. For melt-and-pour and hand-milled soaps, start at about 1 to 3 percent of the soap's total weight.

Scents and Scent Categories

Scent oils, whether fragrance or essential, tend to fall into several broad categories that relate to each other like different parts of an orchestra.

There are no rules to these categories. They are just a starting point for understanding. As you choose scents, learn more about fragrance, and begin creating your own blends (more on that later), you'll be able to connect both intellectually and emotionally with the scents in your soaps.

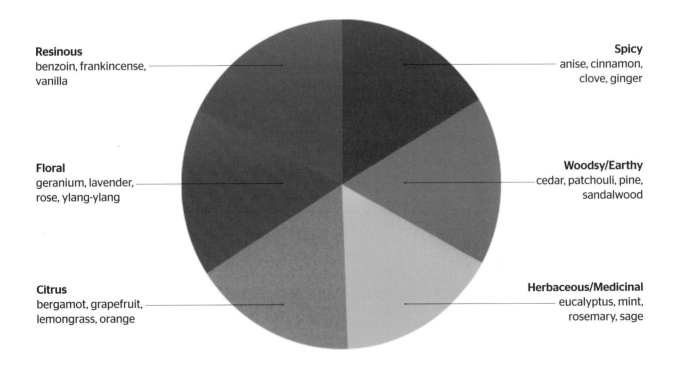

Resinous
benzoin, frankincense, vanilla

Floral
geranium, lavender, rose, ylang-ylang

Citrus
bergamot, grapefruit, lemongrass, orange

Spicy
anise, cinnamon, clove, ginger

Woodsy/Earthy
cedar, patchouli, pine, sandalwood

Herbaceous/Medicinal
eucalyptus, mint, rosemary, sage

Soap Molds

You've likely seen soaps of all shapes and sizes. The molds available to give your soaps their forms range widely—from reused yogurt and milk containers, to cereal and shoeboxes, storage containers, or other baking and cooking ware. Molds can also be made from sections of PVC pipe or corrugated plastic. With found molds, just be sure they

- Have some flexibility or give to them—or (as with PVC pipe) some way for you to get the soap out of the mold easily.

- Will stand up to the soap—if made of porous materials, such as cardboard or wood, you'll need to line the mold with freezer paper (plastic-side up) or a plastic bag.

- Will not react to the soap—be sure there is no aluminum in the mold; it will react to the lye.

There are also many types of molds specifically made for soap, including

1 Single-cavity molds: Usually made from plastic or silicone, these molds make individual soaps in a wide range of themes, shapes, and styles.

2 Loaf molds: Often made of wood (which needs to be lined with freezer paper) or silicone, these molds are great starter molds, allowing you to layer and swirl your batches easily.

3 Slab molds: These molds make the soap in a horizontal slab, usually one, but sometimes two or three bars thick. These molds allow you to swirl the soap and see the swirls. They also often have convenient dividers that allow the soap to be un-molded into individual bars. If made of wood, it also needs to be lined.

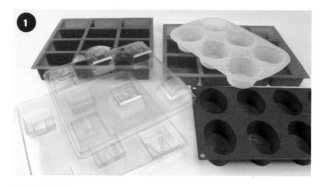

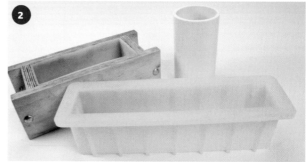

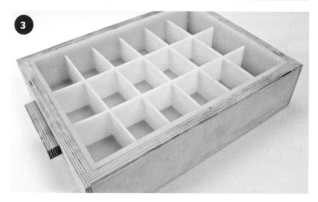

Calculating the Volume of a Soap Mold

Most commercially available soap molds will note their capacity. But homemade molds and, often, single-cavity molds will not have this information, so you will need to calculate the volume of the mold.

For **square or rectangular** molds:

1. Calculate the mold's cubic inches by multiplying the length × width × height to which you will pour the soap. For example: If you have a log mold that is 10 inches (25 cm) long, 2.5 inches (6 cm) wide and 3 inches (7.5 cm) tall, and you plan to fill the mold to the top, multiply 10 × 2.5 × 3 = 75 cubic inches (or 25 × 6 × 7.5 = 1,125 cubic cm).

2. For *imperial measures*, take this total volume and multiply it by 0.4. This gives you the amount of oil in ounces or grams that you should incorporate into the recipe. For example, using the log mold preceding: 75 (the total volume) × 0.4 = 30 ounces of oil.
   To calculate this for *metric*, multiply the total volume by 0.75. or 1,125 × 0.75 = 850 g of oil.

3. Using the percentages of oils in your recipe, calculate each individual oil's amount and use a lye calculator to determine the final recipe for that mold.

For **round or tube** molds:

4. Calculate the volume by multiplying *pi* (3.14) by the radius (half the total width) of the circle squared, and multiply that by the height of the mold. It's not as hard as it sounds. For example: For a 9-inch (23 cm) tube that is 3 inches (7.5 cm) in diameter:
   - The radius is 1.5 inches (3.65 cm). "Squared" is the number multiplied by itself, so 1.5 × 1.5 = 2.25 (or 3.65 × 3.65 = 13.32 cm).
   - *Pi* is a constant generally calculated at 3.14.
   So, for a 3-inch diameter (7.5 cm) PVC tube mold that is 9 inches (23 cm) high, the calculation is 3.14 (*pi*) × 2.25 (radius squared) × 9 (height) = 63.58

or 3.14 [*pi*] × 13.32 [radius squared] × 23 [height] = 962

For *imperial* measurements, multiply the volume by 0.4 to get the amount of oils in the recipe. Example: 63.58 × 0.4 = 25.4 ounces of oils.
For *metric*, multiply the volume by 0.75 or 962 × 0.75 = 721 g of oil.

For **single-cavity or other molds** that are difficult to measure, use the water method.

5. Fill the mold with water and measure that water in **fluid** ounces (ml).

6. Multiply the number of **fluid** ounces of water by 1.8 to get the total cubic inches of the mold. Multiply the ml by 1 to get the total cubic centimeters. For example: A mold holds 10 fluid (295.7 ml) ounces of water: 10 × 1.8 = 18 cubic inches; or 295.7 ml × 1 = 295.7 cubic centimeters.

7. As before, multiply the volume by 0.4 (imperial) or 0.75 (metric) to calculate the amount of oils for that mold. For example: 18 cubic inches × 0.4 = 7.2 ounces of oil in the recipe or 295.7 cubic centimeters × 0.75 = 222 g of oil.

NOTE

These measurements are only approximations, but they are a good starting point to use for nontraditional molds. Even with carefully calculated volumes, and even with standard soap molds, you can sometimes end up with leftover soap. Always keep an additional small mold handy to put any extra soap into.

Hand-Milled Soap

Hand-milled soap is also often called "rebatched" soap—and these two unrelated names embody the two main (also unrelated) benefits of this soap making technique. Whichever name you call it, this method takes a portion of soap, made either by cold or hot process, and grates, chops, or mills it into small shreds. A bit of liquid is added to the shreds and the soap is slowly heated until it melts and reconstitutes into a moldable soap batter. This technique is different than using a melt-and-pour soap base in that the soap used has not been formulated specifically to be melted. *Any soap can be hand milled or rebatched.*

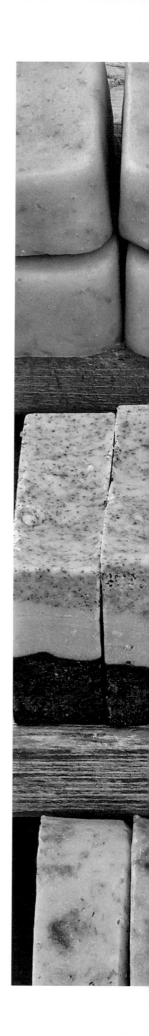

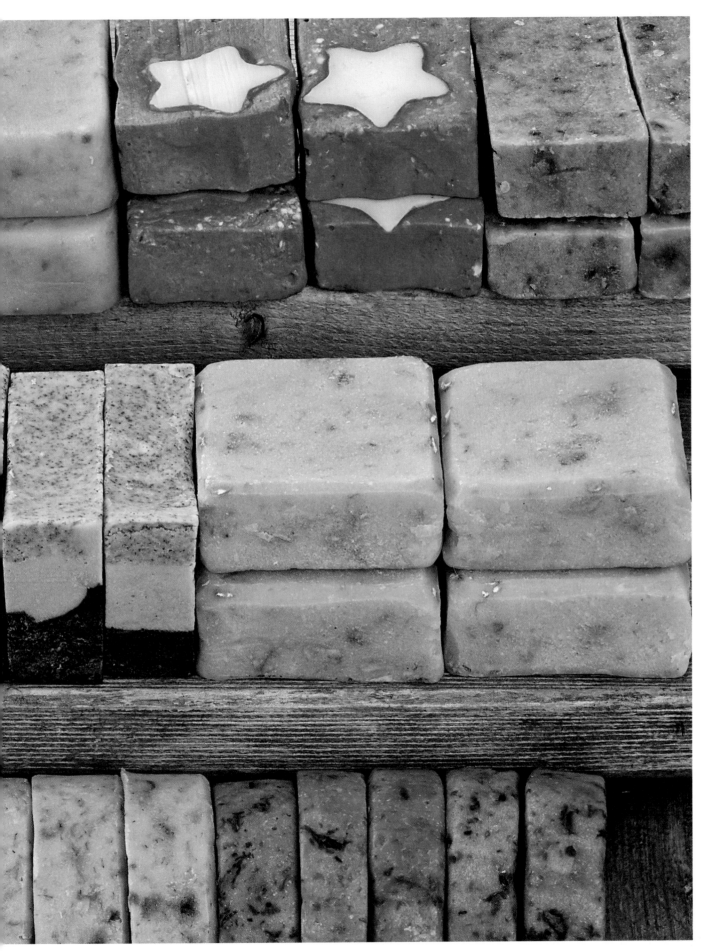

Why Hand Milling?

This technique is called hand milling when it is done intentionally, and there are several benefits and reasons to hand mill a batch of soap.

- Because the soap base is already made, there is no worry about safety issues handling lye.
- As the saponification process has already taken place, delicate fragrances, colors, botanicals, and other additives can be added to the soap without being affected (or destroyed) by the lye.
- Very small batches—even just one bar—can be made using this process. You can make a large batch of uncolored, unscented soap and rebatch portions of it into smaller batches to test fragrances, colors, and other variations you may dream up.

This technique is called rebatching when it is used to rescue, or fix, a batch of soap gone awry in some way.

- If an ingredient (fragrance oil, color, additive) was left out of the original batch of soap, it can be added back in the rebatch.

Is This Really Milled Soap?

Hand-milled soap should not be confused with "French milled," or "triple milled," soap. That centuries-old process grinds, presses, and mills the soap through a large machine several times after it is made. The resulting soap is quite dense, smooth, and uniform in both color and texture. It is wonderful soap, but made through a large-scale mechanical process not easily replicated at home.

- If the soap got too thick suddenly, or separated in the mold, or somehow just didn't go as planned, it can often be redone and saved by rebatching.

The only disadvantage to rebatching is that it's not possible to get the smooth, fluid texture of freshly made soap. Reconstituted hand-milled soap batter is thicker than a new batch of soap, so it needs to be scooped into the molds rather than poured like a new batch. This gives it a much more rustic appearance. Other than that aesthetic challenge, hand milling soap can be a useful technique.

SLOW COOKER METHOD FOR HAND MILLING SOAP

Two things are needed to reconstitute a batch of soap—heat and liquid—and, with both, the key is to add *just enough*.

Heating the Soap

A slow cooker is an effective way to heat soap as it heats slowly and evenly. The soap needs enough heat to remelt, but not so much as to boil or excessively dry it out. A double boiler, or even a low-temperature oven, can be used as well.

Adding the Liquid

How fresh the batch of soap is will determine how much liquid the soap needs to reconstitute. A two-day-old batch will need hardly any liquid, whereas a two-week- or two-month-old batch will need more. The soap should be thoroughly moist, but not dripping. A good starting point with a relatively fresh batch of soap is 2 to 3 ounces (57 to 85 g) of liquid per 1 pound (454 g) of soap.

Cow's milk or goat's milk is the most common liquid added to hand-milled soap because it helps the soap melt more easily and improves the smoothness and fluidity immensely. But a variety of liquids can be used, including plain water, and even liquids such as juice, tea, and other plant-based milks such as coconut, soy, or almond.

Though any slow, even heat source will work, a slow cooker is the easiest method to rebatch soap in, as the soap is easily visible and stirrable.

HAND-MILLED OATMEAL AND ROSE CLAY SOAPS

1 Place the grated soap shreds (A) in the slow cooker (B). Add the liquid and stir to moisten the soap shreds evenly. Turn the cooker to low heat.

2 After 20 to 30 minutes, check the soap. The bottom layer will have started to melt and turn translucent. Gently stir the soap to remix it. After 20 to 30 minutes more, check and stir the soap again. It will be smoother, but will still contain some chunks. Scrape off any soap bits stuck to the side of the slow cooker (C).

3 After another 20 to 30 minutes, the soap should be evenly smooth (D).

4 Separate the batch into two measuring cups. To one cup, stir in half the fragrance oil and the oatmeal (E). To the other, stir in the remaining fragrance oil, clay, and rose petals. (Note: These two soaps are scented with the same fragrance; use two different fragrances, if desired.)

5 Scoop the soap into the mold and set it aside to cool and harden (F). Depending on how much liquid is used, it may take two to three days for it to harden enough to remove it from the mold.

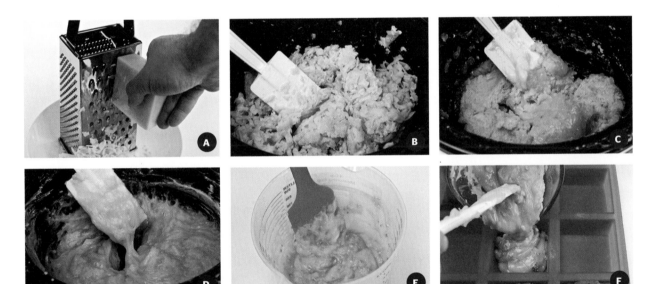

INGREDIENTS
- 1 lb (454 g) grated soap
- 2 to 3 ounces (57 to 85 g) liquid of choice

ADDITIVES
- 0.5 ounce (14 g) fragrance oil or essential oil, divided
- 1 tablespoon (5 g) oatmeal (for half the batch)
- 1 teaspoon rose clay (for the other half batch
- 1 tablespoon (1.5 g) rose petals (for the other half batch)

EQUIPMENT
- Slow cooker
- Basic soap-making equipment (see page 14)

Makes about 1 pound (454 g)

OVEN-ROASTING BAG METHOD FOR HAND MILLING SOAP

The development of plastic oven-roasting bags made rebatching soap even easier than in a slow cooker. The soap is easily visible and the water provides very even heating of the soap. Instead of stirring, you mix it by squishing the soap around in the bag.

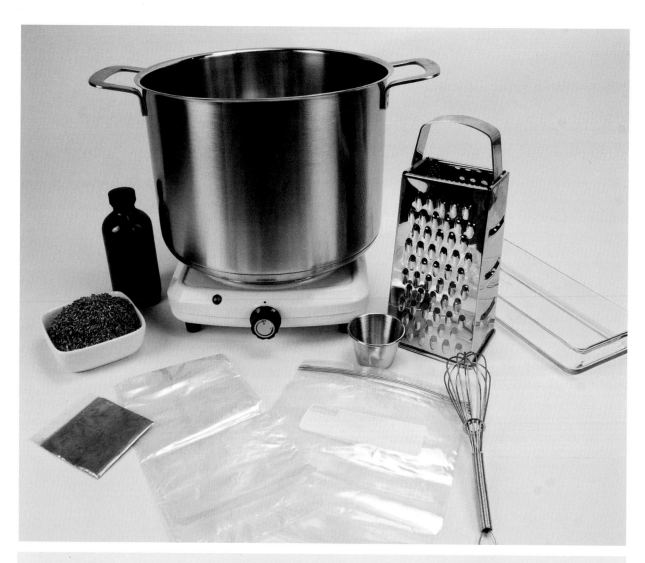

INGREDIENTS

- 1 lb (454 g) grated soap
- 2 to 3 ounces (57 to 85 g) liquid of choice

Makes about 1 pound (454 g)

ADDITIVES

- 0.5 ounce (14 g) fragrance oil or essential oil
- 2 tablespoons (4 g) lavender buds
- ½ teaspoon blue-green mica

EQUIPMENT

- Large plastic oven-roasting bag
- Large pot of water at a medium simmer
- Basic soap-making equipment (see page 14)

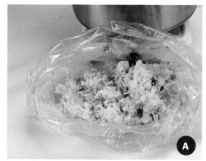

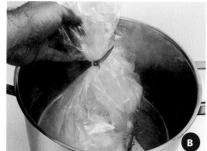

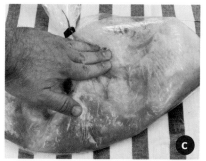

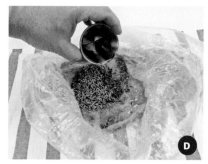

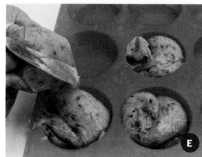

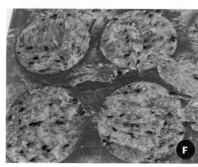

HAND MILLED LAVENDAR SOAP

1 Place the grated soap shreds into the oven-roasting bag. Add the liquid and seal the bag tightly. Squish the soap shreds and liquid together to mix evenly and moisten the shreds (A).

2 Place the bag into the pot of simmering water (B). After 20 to 30 minutes, remove the bag and check the soap. As with the slow cooker method, the soap will have started to melt and turn translucent. Squish the soap around in the bag to mix it (C). The soap will be hot so you might want to wear oven mitts. Return the soap to the simmering water.

3 After 20 to 30 minutes more, check and mix the soap again to ensure it is being evenly heated.

4 After another 20 to 30 minutes, the soap should be evenly melted. Remove the bag of soap from the pot. Carefully add the fragrance oil, lavender buds, and mica to the bag (D). Seal the bag and thoroughly mix the soap again.

5 Cut off a bottom corner of the bag and squeeze the soap into the mold (E).

6 With a rubber spatula, smooth the top and set the soap aside to cool and harden. Depending on how much liquid is used, it may take two to three days for the soap to harden enough to remove it from the mold (F).

Hand-Milled Soap Recipes

Any of these recipes can be made using either the slow cooker or oven-roasting bag method. They all start with 1 to 2 pounds (454 to 908 g) freshly grated soap, but can easily be scaled to make larger batches.

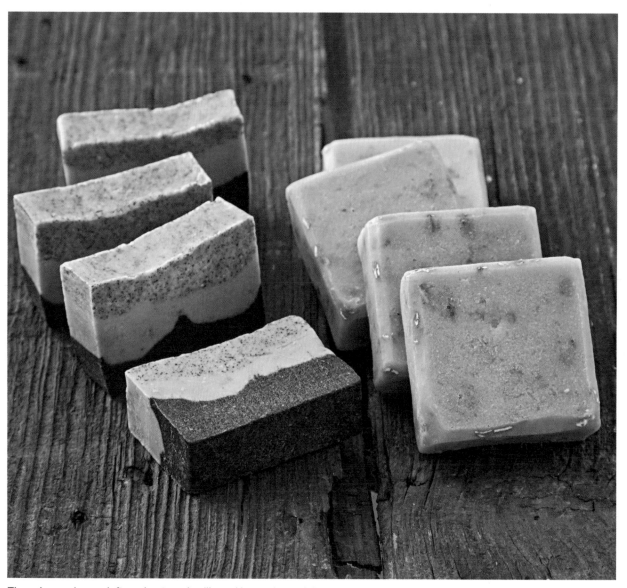

Three-layered soap, left, and oatmeal, milk, and honey bars, right.

INGREDIENTS

- 1 lb (454 g) grated soap
- 2 to 3 ounces (57 to 85 g) goat's milk or cow's milk

ADDITIVES

- 0.5 ounce (14 g) fragrance oil or essential oil
- 2 tablespoons (10 g) lightly ground oatmeal
- 1 tablespoon (20 g) honey

EQUIPMENT

- Basic soap-making equipment (see page 14)

Makes about 1 pound (454 g)

OATMEAL, MILK, AND HONEY BAR

This naturally colored bar is lightly exfoliating with the additional natural soothing benefits of milk and honey.

1 Stir the goat's milk into the shreds and melt the soap using slow cooker or roasting bag method.

2 When fully melted, stir in the fragrance oil and oatmeal.

3 Lightly drizzle the honey over the soap to help disperse it evenly.

4 Mix the soap well and scoop it into the mold and set aside to cool and harden.

THREE-LAYERED SOAP

This soap incorporates clay, activated charcoal, and ground walnut shells into a cleansing and exfoliating bar that is molded in a small (2 pounds or 908 g) loaf mold.

INGREDIENTS

- 28 ounces (794 g) grated soap
- 4 to 6 ounces (113 to 170 g) liquid of choice

ADDITIVES

- 1 ounce (14 g) fragrance oil or essential oil
- 1 to 2 tablespoons (5 to 10 g) ground walnut shells
- 1 tablespoon (9 g) kaolin, bentonite, or French green clay
- 1 teaspoon activated charcoal—a little goes a long way

EQUIPMENT

- Basic soap-making equipment (see page 14)

Makes about 2 pounds (907 g)

1 Stir the liquid into the shreds and melt the soap using slow cooker or oven roasting bag method.

2 When fully melted, stir in the fragrance oil. Separate the mixture into three portions.

3 Into the first portion, mix the walnut shells. Into the second portion, blend the clay. Into the third portion, add the charcoal.

4 Layer each portion in the mold. For a flatter look to the layers, gently scoop or pour the soap into the mold and smooth each layer afterward. Set aside to cool and harden.

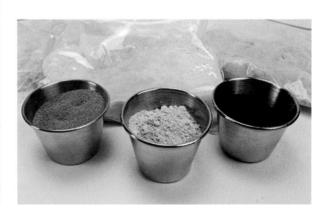

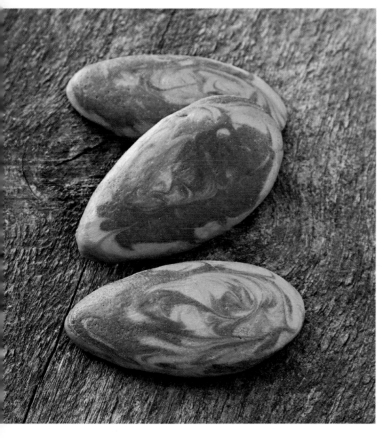

SWIRLED HAND-MILLED SOAP BARS

Some swirling is possible with hand-milled soap, especially if the soap is not very old and has had sodium lactate added. This technique can be done in a loaf or log mold or in individual molds.

INGREDIENTS
- 1 lb (454 g) fresh grated soap
- 2 to 3 ounces (57 to 85 g) liquid of choice
- 1 ounce (28 g) sodium lactate

ADDITIVES
- 0.5 ounce (14 g) fragrance oil or essential oil
- ½ teaspoon yellow mica
- ½ teaspoon red mica
- ½ teaspoon purple mica

EQUIPMENT
- Basic soap-making equipment (see page 14)
- Chopstick

Makes about 1 pound (454 g)

1 Stir the liquid into the shreds and melt the soap using slow cooker or oven-roasting bag method. When fully melted, separate the batch into three portions.

2 Add the yellow mica to one portion, the red mica to the second portion, and the purple mica to the third. Mix each well (A).

3 Spoon or pour a small bit of each color into the mold(s), laying one color next to the other, and on top of the other (B).

4 When the molds are filled, use a chopstick to swirl the soap. In addition to swirling side to side, push the chopstick all the way to the bottom of the mold to get the colors on the bottom swirled up to the top (C). Set aside to cool and harden.

This swirl technique works best in larger molds, such as loaf/log molds, but (as shown) it can be done in individual molds, as well. With individual molds, you may need to shave or wash the top layer (the bottom of the mold cavity) to reveal the swirls.

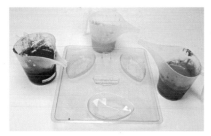
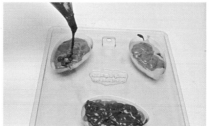
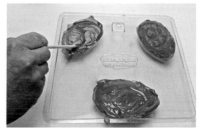

DOUBLE ROSE HAND-MILLED SOAP

Rose clay and rose petals give this soap (shown near right) a lovely old-fashioned look. You can substitute other colorants or botanicals as well.

1 Stir the liquid into the shreds and melt the soap using slow cooker or oven-roasting bag method. When fully melted, add the rose clay and mix well. Clays tend to clump and create specs in the soap. Premixing it into the liquid glycerin (if using) helps the clay disperse more evenly.

2 Gently mix in the rose petals.

3 Scoop the soap into the mold and set aside to cool and harden.

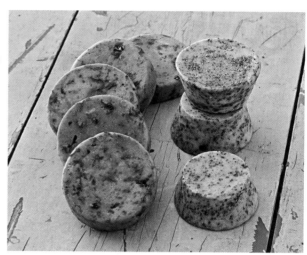

INGREDIENTS
- 1 lb (454 g) grated soap
- 2 to 3 ounces (57 to 85 g) liquid of choice

ADDITIVES
- 0.5 ounce (14 g) fragrance oil or essential oil
- 1 tablespoon (15 g) rose clay
- 2 tablespoons (30 ml) liquid glycerin (optional)
- 1 tablespoon (1.5 g) lightly crushed rose petals buds

EQUIPMENT
- Basic soap-making equipment (see page 14)

Makes about 1 pound (454 g)

SCRUBBY GARDENER'S SOAP

This soap (above at far right) uses extra-scrubby exfoliants and a strong essential oil blend to clean even the dirtiest hands. Other fragrance oils or essential oils can be substituted, as can other exfoliants, for those called for here.

1 Stir the liquid into the shreds and melt the soap using slow cooker or oven-roasting bag method. When fully melted, add the essential oil blend and pumice and mix well.

2 Add the sandalwood powder and poppy seeds. Mix lightly, which creates a slightly variegated, or swirled, look.

3 Scoop the soap into the mold and set aside to cool and harden.

INGREDIENTS
- 1 lb (454 g) grated soap
- 2 to 3 ounces (57 to 85 g) liquid of choice

ADDITIVES
- 0.5 ounce (14 g) essential oil blend, consisting of
  - 0.2 ounce (5.5 g) lavender essential oil
  - 0.1 ounce (2.8 g) eucalyptus essential oil
  - 0.1 ounce (2.8 g) tea tree essential oil
  - 0.1 ounce (2.8 g) clove essential oil
  - 1 tablespoon (9.5 g) pumice
- 1 tablespoon (6 g) red sandalwood powder
- 1 tablespoon (9 g) poppy seeds

EQUIPMENT
- Basic soap-making equipment (see page 14)

Makes about 1 pound (454 g)

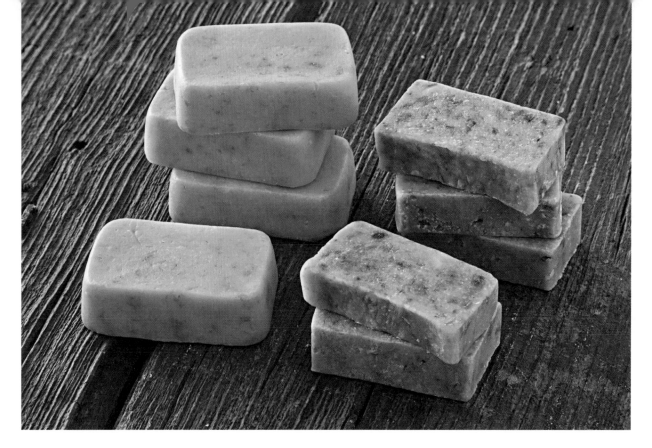

GARDEN OF GREENS SOAP

This soap (above right) takes advantage of one prime benefit of hand-milled soap: The spinach and kale would turn black when exposed to lye in a cold process bar, but hand milling this batch allows them to retain their natural green color. Using water instead of milk helps keep the soap a bit whiter and retain a bit of the bright green color as well. The spirulina powder gives a natural green color (mica could also be used) throughout to complement the dark green botanicals.

INGREDIENTS
- 3 tablespoons (3.75 g) crushed, dried spinach leaves
- 3 tablespoons (1.8 g) crushed, dried kale leaves
- 28 ounces (794 g) grated soap
- 4 to 6 ounces (113 to 170 g) water

ADDITIVES
- 1 ounce (14 g) fragrance oil or essential oil
- 1 teaspoon spirulina powder or green mica

EQUIPMENT
- Basic soap-making equipment (see page 14)

Makes about 2 pounds (907 g)

1 Bake a few handfuls of fresh spinach and kale leaves in a low (200°F or 93°C) oven until fully dried, about 30 minutes. Lightly crush the leaves and set aside.

2 Stir the liquid into the shreds and melt the soap using slow cooker or oven roasting bag method.

3 When fully melted, add the fragrance oil and spirulina and mix well.

4 Add the spinach and kale leaves last and mix gently.

5 Scoop the soap into the mold and set aside to cool and harden.

INGREDIENTS

- 3 tablespoons (20.25 g) dried lemon, orange, or lime peel (see step 1)
- 1 lb (454 g) grated soap
- 2 to 3 ounces (57 to 85 g) liquid of choice

ADDITIVES

- 0.5 ounce (14 g) essential oil blend, consisting of:
  - 0.2 ounce (5.5 g) orange essential oil
  - 0.1 ounce (2.8 g) lemon essential oil
  - 0.1 ounce (2.8 g) litsea cubeba essential oil

EQUIPMENT

- Basic soap-making equipment (see page 14)

Makes about 1 pound (454 g)

CITRUS PEEL SOAP

This soap, like the Garden of Greens soap (opposite page), also takes advantage of the hand-milling method that keeps the citrus peels from turning black after being exposed to lye. The peels are lightly exfoliating and the orange color comes naturally from the essential oils.

1. Finely grate 3 tablespoons (20.25 g) citrus peel (just the outer, colored layer) and set aside to dry for a few days.

2. Stir the liquid into the shreds and melt the soap using slow cooker or oven roasting bag method.

3. When fully melted, add the essential oils and citrus peel. Mix well.

4. Scoop the soap into the mold and set aside to cool and harden.

FLOWER PETALS SOAP

Most any choice and combination of flower petals can be used in this pretty soap, as they won't be turned black by contact with lye. Avoid any petals that could irritate the skin or are too scratchy.

1. Stir the liquid into the shreds and melt the soap using slow cooker or oven-roasting bag method. When fully melted, thoroughly mix in the fragrance oil, flower petals, and yellow mica.

2. Scoop the soap into the mold and set aside to cool and harden.

INGREDIENTS

- 1 lb (454 g) grated soap
- 2 to 3 ounces (57 to 85 g) liquid of choice

ADDITIVES

- 0.5 ounce (14 g) fragrance oil or essential oil
- 2 to 3 tablespoons (4 to 6 g) lightly crushed flower petals, such as calendula, lavender, or chamomile
- ½ teaspoon yellow mica

EQUIPMENT

- Basic soap-making equipment (see page 14)

Makes about 1 pound (454 g)

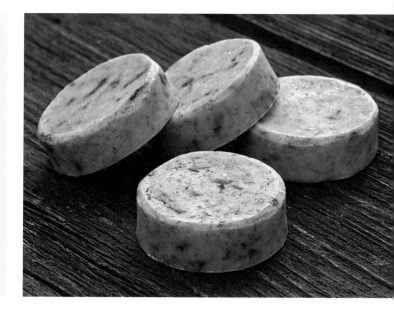

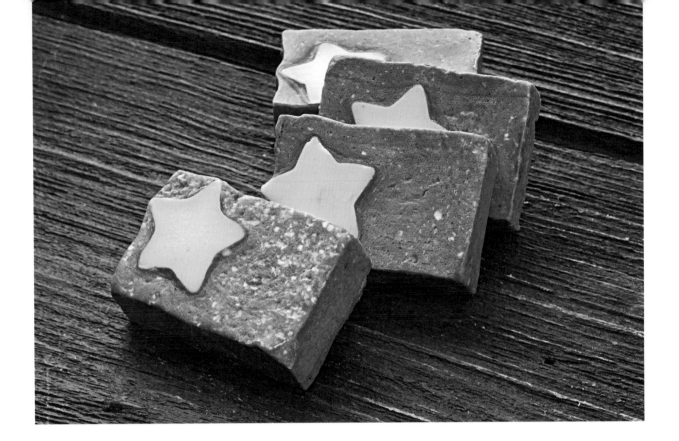

STARRY NIGHT SOAP

This soap uses a star-shaped piece of soap embedded into the bar. This "embed" can be made from hand-milled, melt-and-pour, or cold process soap molded in a star-shaped tube mold or cut out with a star-shaped cookie cutter. The overall stars effect in the bar comes from the very finely grated, well-dried soap. If you don't have a well-cured bar of white soap to grate, a purchased bar of white soap works very well.

1 Place the star embed into the mold cavity and sprinkle a light layer of grated white soap around the star.

2 Stir the liquid into the shreds and melt the soap using slow cooker or oven-roasting bag method. When fully melted, mix in the fragrance oil, blue mica, and remaining grated white soap.

3 Gently scoop the blue soap into the mold cavities, being careful not to move the star embed and surrounding white shreds too much. When finished pouring, reposition the star, if necessary. Set aside to cool and harden.

4 When the soap is fully hardened, you may need to plane or wash off the top layer of soap to reveal the star embed and surrounding white stars.

INGREDIENTS
- Star embed
- 3 tablespoons (45 g) finely grated, well-cured, dried white soap
- 1 lb (454 g) grated fresh soap
- 2 to 3 ounces (57 to 85 g) liquid of choice

ADDITIVES
- 0.5 ounce (14 g) fragrance oil or essential oil
- 1 teaspoon blue mica

EQUIPMENT
- Basic soap-making equipment (see page 14)

Makes about 1 pound (454 g)

Hand-Milled Soap:
Tips and Troubleshooting

Hand-milled soap will never look like freshly poured cold process soap or commercially milled soaps, but here are a few tips to help make the best soap possible.

Tips for Hand Milling or Rebatching Soap

1 The sooner you can mill or rebatch the soap after it is first made, the easier it will be to remelt and the less liquid you will need to add.

2 Use enough liquid to reconstitute. The more you add, the more that will have to evaporate, and the more your soap may shrink or warp.

3 Use milk. Milk, whether fresh, canned, or powdered, will make the soap reconstitute and be much more fluid. It can give the soap a bit of an ivory color, though, so take that into account when creating your recipe.

4 Go slowly. The more slowly and evenly you heat the shredded soap, the better. Heating it too quickly can cause it to dry and scorch.

5 If you have extra time, add the liquid to the shreds and let sit overnight. The soap will absorb the liquid and begin to soften before it is heated—especially helpful with older soap.

6 If you're rebatching to save a batch you left an ingredient out of, only do so if you know *exactly* what that ingredient is. For example, if you left out an oil and you know which oil it is (and how much of it), it can be added back into the batch. But if you mismeasured and don't know by how much, you're just guessing and the batch may not be able to be saved. This is especially important if you mismeasured the lye.

Using Sodium Lactate

Sodium lactate is a salt derived from lactic acid and sold in liquid form by many soap-making suppliers. When used in a very fresh—less than two-week-old—batch of soap, it makes the soap batter amazingly more fluid and pourable, almost as pourable as fresh cold process soap. If your soap is still very soft and fresh, add between 0.5 and 1 ounce (14 to 28 g) per 1 pound (454 g) of soap shreds along with the other liquids to improve the soap's fluidity. Unfortunately, its effect seems to diminish as the batch of soap gets older.

Troubleshooting Hand-Milled Soap

1 **The soap is too lumpy.** Rebatched soap will not have the same smoothness as a fresh batch of soap, even when adding milk or sodium lactate.

2 **The soap is too soft.** Adding too much liquid may make your soap pour better and be less lumpy, but it will take much longer to dry and harden. The only cure for this is time.

3 **My soap is shrinking/changing shape as it dries.** All the water you add to the shreds needs to evaporate, causing the soap to shrink. Turn the soap every few days so the liquid evaporates evenly.

4 **My colorants or additives aren't blended evenly in the soap.** Some additives are more difficult to blend evenly into rebatched soap. Premixing with a bit of glycerin or the liquid you're using can help—especially with clays and powdered colorants.

Melt-and-Pour Soap

Although some may say it is just for beginners, or not real soap, melt-and-pour soap is a simple and wonderful way to create your own handmade soaps. The melt-and-pour soap base is made like all soap, with lye and oils, but with additional ingredients that help it melt easily when heated.

Because you don't have to deal with recipe calculation or worry about handling lye, it's a very simple and safe way to make soap. Think of it like a basic "just add water" cake mix. It is perfectly useable as is, but you can add extra ingredients, or decorations, or bake it in a certain way, to make it exactly how you want it.

Because you aren't creating the soap from scratch, using a melt-and-pour base allows you to focus on your soap's design—its scent, color, and shape—and customization. Whether adding simple color, fragrance, or botanical additives, or complex multilayered designs, the transparent and quick-hardening nature of melt-and-pour soap allows for designs that aren't possible in soap made from scratch.

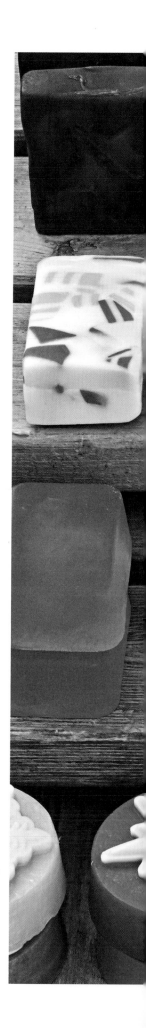

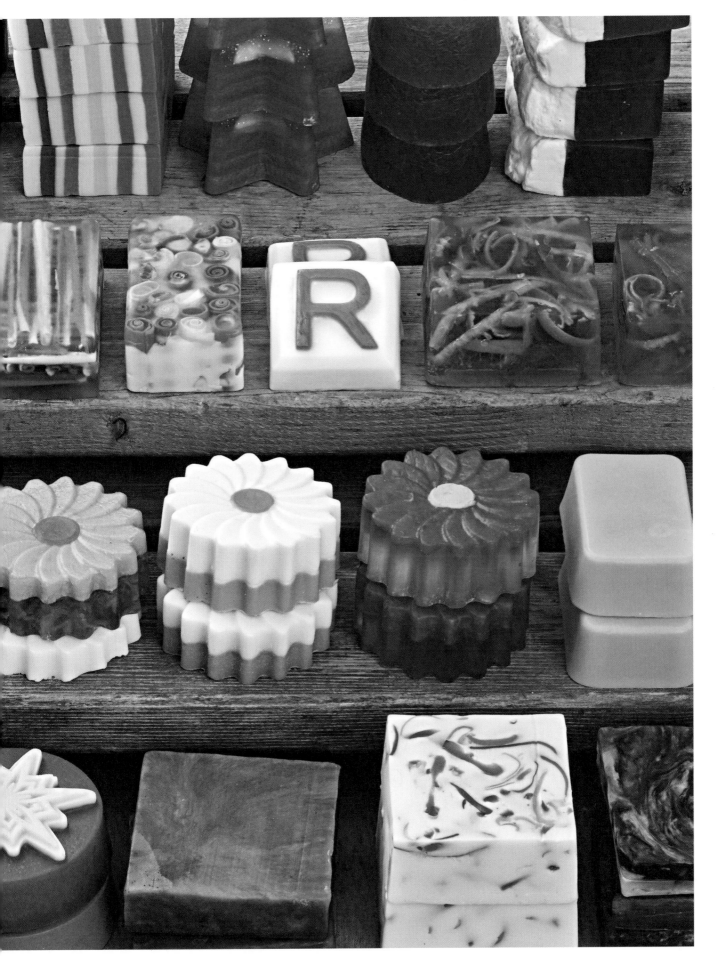

Types of Melt-and-Pour Bases

Soap making suppliers carry a number of melt-and-pour bases—from specialty to the very basic. The different bases bring different qualities to your finished soaps.

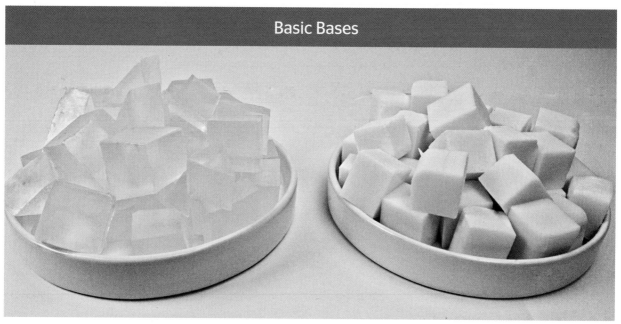

Basic Bases

Clear melt-and-pour base (left) and white melt-and-pour base (right).

Remember, all soap contains these basic ingredients—*lye (sodium hydroxide), water, and oils*. Melt-and-pour soap is the same. On the ingredient list for your soap base, you are likely to see ingredients such as, "water, coconut oil, palm oil, and sodium hydroxide" or "sodium laurate and sodium stearate." The former is the list of ingredients *before* the ingredients are mixed. The latter is the list of ingredients *after* they are transformed into soap by the saponification process.

In addition to the lye, water, and oils, other ingredients are added to the base to allow it to melt, make it lather, or add other custom attributes. Some additional ingredients you are likely to see are

- **Glycerin and sorbitol** (a sugar-derived alcohol) help make the soap base transparent.

- **Propylene glycol** (a common solvent widely used in many foods and cosmetics) helps the soap melt.

- **Sodium laureth sulfate** (SLeS) or sodium lauryl sulfate (SLS); detergents, foaming agents, and surfactants) helps the soap lather, clean, and rinse well.

You may also see ingredients such as titanium dioxide, which makes the soap base white, as well as honey, aloe, shea butter, goat's milk, or oatmeal. These ingredients provide moisturizing and other benefits for the skin as well as label appeal.

Specialty Bases

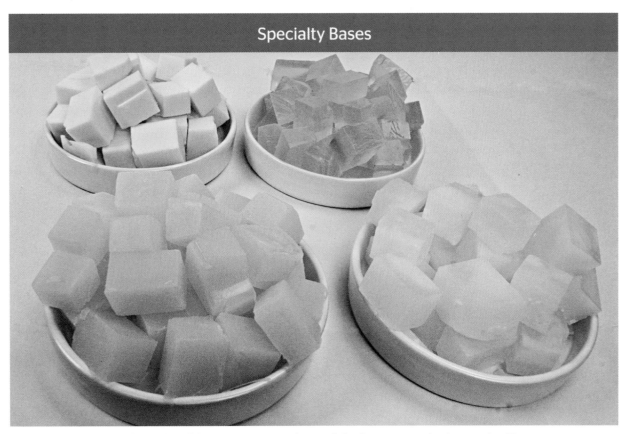

Clockwise from upper left: goat's milk base; carrot, cucumber, and aloe base; suspension base; natural base.

In addition to the bases with special additives, there are also bases formulated for special purposes. Some of the most common are

- **Suspension base:** A much thicker base that helps additives stay suspended in the melted soap rather than sinking to the bottom.

- **Low-sweat base:** Formulated to mimic cold process soap more closely, a low-sweat base has a lower glycerin content so it is less prone to sweating like standard melt-and-pour soaps.

- **Natural base:** A base formulated without any detergents or surfactants to be as natural as possible.

- **Special ingredient base:** Many specialty bases are available with special ingredients such as aloe, goat's milk, cucumber, honey, shea butter, hemp oil, and more.

Regardless of the base you use, melt-and-pour soap allows you to just melt the soap, add your color, fragrance, and additives, and pour it into a mold. It's ready to use as soon as it cools and hardens.

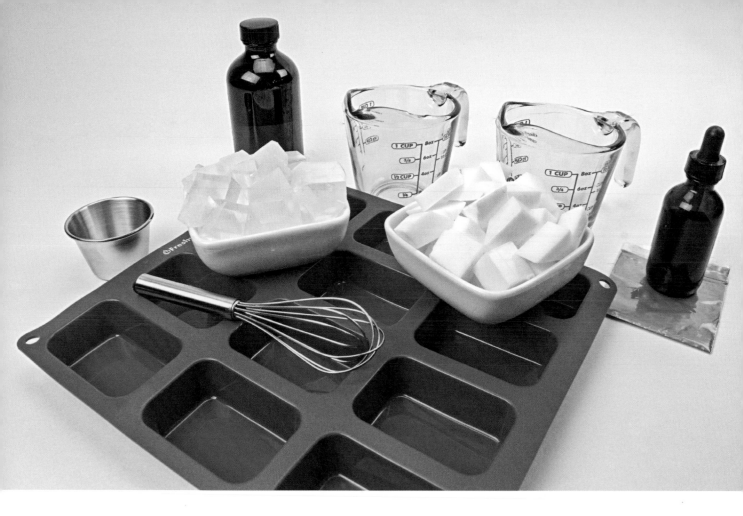

Customizing Your Melt-and-Pour Soap

Like all recipes, you can customize your melt-and-pour soap with scent, color, and many other additives.

Adding Fragrance

Multiplying the soap base weight by 3 percent is a good starting point for determining the amount of fragrance to add. That equals about 0.5 ounce (14 g) per 1 pound (454 g) of soap base. This can be adjusted based on the strength of your fragrance. Use a bit more if the fragrance is light; less if the fragrance is strong. Add the fragrance after the soap melts, and gently stir to mix it in.

Fragrance tips:

• Although you can use either fragrance oils or essential oils, be sure they are safe to use in soap.

• Adding the fragrance oil into the melted soap is likely to make it cloudy, at first. Keep stirring for 20 to 30 seconds and it should clear.

Adding Color

Melt-and-pour soaps can use the same range of natural and synthetic colorants as other soaps. Add them after the soap melts and gently stir to mix them in.

A few color tips:

• Rich or dark colors work best in a clear soap base. White soap bases give a more pastel color.

- Dyes or water-based colorants allow for wonderful transparent effects, but the colors will bleed over time.

- Some colorants, such as clays and oxides, disperse much better if you premix them in a bit of glycerin before adding them to your soap.

- Colorants that may shift or morph in cold process soap (due to its high pH) work just fine in melt-and-pour soaps.

- Take your fragrance oil's or essential oil's color into account when creating your recipe. Also, vanilla-containing fragrances will cause your soap to turn brown to some degree.

Other Additives

Like all soap recipes, you can add custom ingredients to create exfoliating or moisturizing qualities, or just visual appeal. One great benefit of melt-and-pour soap is the saponification process is complete, so anything you add will not be affected by the lye. This allows the use of botanicals, such as flower petals, that would normally turn black from exposure to the lye.

Additive tips:

- Remember that whatever you put into the soap, will eventually come out of the soap in the shower or tub.

- Heavier additives can settle to the bottom of the mold. To address this, pour the soap at a lower temperature when the soap is thicker, or use a specialty suspension base (see page 41).

Basic Method for Making Melt-and-Pour Soap

Follow these ten steps for perfect soaps.

1 Start with your preferred melt-and-pour soap base. Cut up and weigh enough soap to make the number of bars you want, with a little extra for waste allowance. The smaller and more uniform the soap chunks are, the more quickly and evenly they will melt.

2 Put the soap chunks into a heatproof container and melt them in the microwave in 30- to 45-second bursts, stirring in between. The soap will begin to melt at about 120°F to 130°F (49°C to 54.5°C).

3 Keep heating and melting *slowly*. Watch the soap carefully to make sure it does not start to boil. Continue melting and stirring in 30- to 45-second bursts until the soap is almost completely melted. The last remaining soap chunks should melt as you stir the soap and add the other ingredients. If not, give the soap another 5 to 10 seconds in the microwave to finish the melting, or just remove the unmelted chunks.

4 While the soap melts, weigh the fragrance oil. You will need about 3 percent of the soap's total weight. This batch makes 1 pound (454 g) of soap or four 4-ounce (115 g) bars, so use 0.5 ounce (14 g) fragrance oil.
(continued)

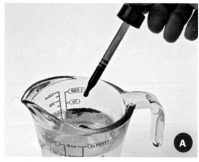
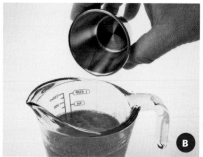
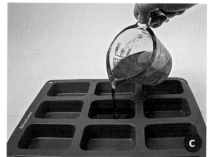
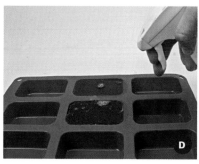
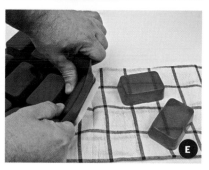

5 When the soap is fully melted, stir in the colorant, being careful not to create too many bubbles in the soap (A).

6 Once the melted soap cools to about 130°F (55°C), gently stir in the fragrance oil (B).

7 Once all additives are stirred in, it is time to pour the soap into the molds. If the soap begins to thicken too much to pour smoothly, reheat it for a few seconds to make it more fluid (C).

8 Lightly spray the soap with rubbing alcohol to remove any bubbles that may have formed (D).

9 Let the soap sit, cool, and harden. This should take an hour or so. To speed the process, it's okay to refrigerate the soap. But just like a glass of cold water, the soap may sweat.

10 As soon as the soap cools and hardens, it's ready to unmold and use (E).

What Is the Order of Ingredients?

Once the soap melts, the fragrance, color, and any other ingredients can be added in any order. However, some fragrance oils and additives can also affect the soap's color. Adding the fragrance oil first allows you to see how its color may affect the soap's color before you add the colorants. Adding any other additives (such as botanicals) last, allows the soap to cool as much as possible, helping keep the additives suspended.

Layered Melt-and-Pour Designs

Because it cools and hardens so quickly, melt-and-pour soap allows for easy layering. Many single-cavity mold designs have raised areas that lend themselves to pouring or piping in the melted soap with a plastic pipette. The key when piping the soap into the mold is to keep it hot and fluid, about 150°F (65.5°C). This technique and these molds allow you to create layered, multicolor, custom designs easily.

Basic Layered Soaps with Piped-in Designs

1 Melt 1 to 2 ounces (28 to 56 g) soap base and add a nonbleeding colorant or mica, if desired.

2 With the soap still hot and fluid (about 150°F or 65.5°C), draw the soap into the pipette and pipe the soap into the desired section of the mold (A).

3 Lightly spray the soap with rubbing alcohol to remove any bubbles.

4 Let the piped soap cool and harden.

5 Melt and color the soap for the bottom of the soap bar.

6 Lightly spray the first piped soap with rubbing alcohol. This helps the layers adhere to each other better.

7 When the second pour of soap cools to about 130°F (54.5°C), pour it into the mold (B).

8 Let the soap cool and harden and gently unmold it (C). With silicone molds, the soap pops out easily. With plastic molds, use both thumbs to firmly, but slowly, press the soap out of the mold. Refrigerating the soap for 15 to 20 minutes helps the soap release from the mold, as well.

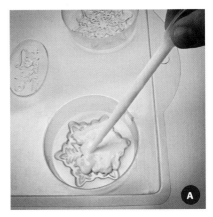 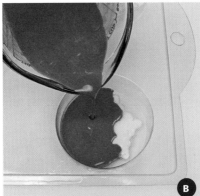 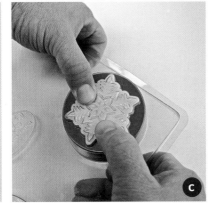

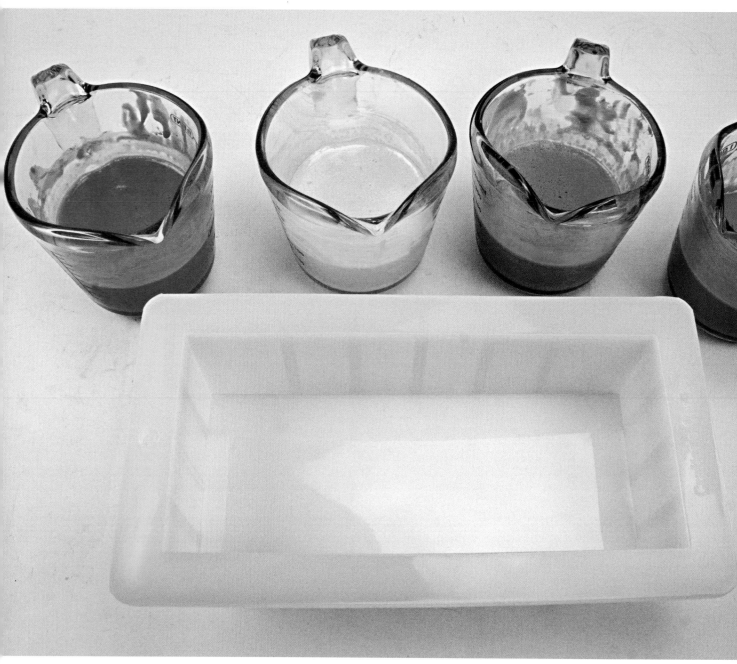

Four portions of colored melt-and-pour soap for a five-layered soap bar.

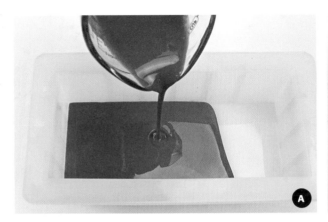

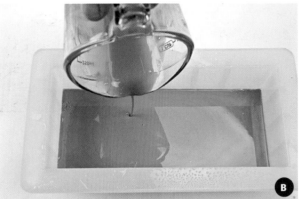

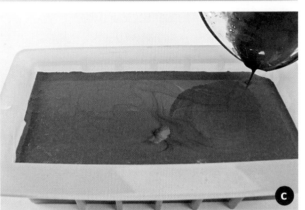

Melt-and-Pour Soap with Multiple Layers

This soap uses the same basic layering technique as the piped-in design (see page 45), but is, instead, made in multiple layers in a larger loaf-style mold. This mold holds about two pounds (908 g) of soap. The soap (as shown) has five layers: one layer each of five colors.

1 Melt 3 ounces (85 g) white soap base and add about ⅛ teaspoon blue mica. Stir gently to mix in the colorant thoroughly. Pour the first layer into the mold (A). Let it cool and harden for 20 to 30 minutes.

2 Melt 3 ounces (85 g) white soap base and add about ⅛ teaspoon pink mica. Lightly spray the first layer with rubbing alcohol and pour in the second layer (B). Temperature is important here. You want the second layer to be about 130°F (54.5°C)—warm enough to pour evenly, but cool enough not to melt the first layer. Repeat this step with the third color.

3 Repeat step 2 for the remaining layers until the mold is full (C).

4 When the soap is completely cooled and hardened, unmold it and slice it with a sharp knife.

Embedding Botanicals

In addition to fragrance and color, natural botanicals can be added to your melt-and-pour soaps. They can add natural color, exfoliation, or just aesthetic interest. As the soap base is already made, additives that don't stand up to contact with the lye work well in melt-and-pour soap.

There are a few methods to add botanicals to your soap.

Mixing Botanicals Throughout

This is the simplest way to mix in botanicals, but the melted soap's fluid nature means heavier additives sink to the bottom of the mold. To help keep them evenly mixed, wait until the soap thickens a bit (to about 120°F or 49°C) or use a suspension base (see page 41).

1 Chop, weigh, and melt your soap base.

2 Stir in the fragrance oil and color, if desired.

3 Stir in the botanicals. If using a suspension base, pour at 130°F (54.5°C) or so. If using a standard base, keep stirring gently until the soap cools to between 105°F and 110°F (40.5°C and 43°C) to pour into the mold.

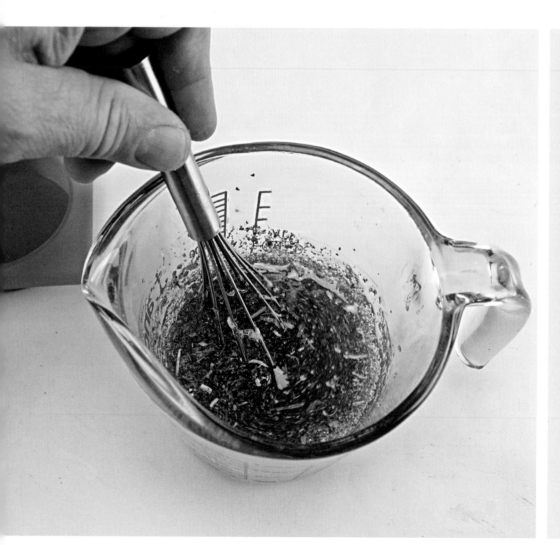

Botanicals and Color Bleed

Just like liquid dyes, many botanicals can cause color bleed in melt-and-pour soap. Coffee grounds, mint leaves, and some flower petals—anything you can make a tea from—will bleed color. One way to minimize this is to brew the botanicals. Use already brewed coffee grounds or make a tea using your leaves or flower petals first. Let them dry completely and use them in your soap.

Letting the Botanicals Settle

This method allows the botanicals to settle on purpose, creating a top layer of interest. With white soap bases, this is best accomplished by mixing the botanicals into the melted soap and pouring it while still hot and fluid (about 140°F or 60°C). With clear soap bases, you can also sprinkle the additive into the mold first and layer the soap on top of the botanicals.

*If using a **clear** base:*

1 Sprinkle a layer of botanicals into your soap molds first.

2 Chop, weigh, and melt your soap base.

3 Stir in the fragrance oil and color, if desired.

4 Use a chopstick to redistribute the botanicals that shifted during the pouring (A).

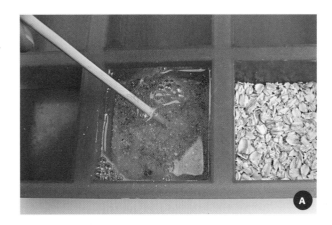

*If using a **white** base:*

1 Stir the botanicals into the hot soap base.

2 Pour the soap into the molds.

Layering the Botanicals

Pouring the soap into the mold in layers can distribute the botanicals evenly throughout the bar and create marvelous visual effects as well, especially in clear soap bases. Multiple layers can be created with multiple additives or just one distributed throughout the bar. Using all clear soap base gives a stained glass, or amber, effect. Adding a white layer on the bottom provides a bright backdrop that makes the botanicals' colors pop.

1 Chop, weigh, and melt the soap base.

2 Stir in the fragrance oil and color, if desired.

3 Pour a thin (0.25 inch or 6 mm) layer of clear soap in the bottom of the mold. Cover the remaining melted soap with plastic wrap and set it aside in a warm place. Let the first layer cool and harden.

4 Warm the remaining soap base to about 130°F (54.5°C).

5 Lightly spray the first layer with rubbing alcohol.

6 Sprinkle the first layer of botanicals into the mold (A).

7 Pour enough melted soap to cover the botanicals. Use a chopstick to rearrange them so they are distributed the way you want.

8 Set aside the remaining soap base as before, and let the second layer cool and harden.

9 Lightly spray the second layer with rubbing alcohol and sprinkle a second layer of botanicals into the mold.

10 Warm the soap base to about 130°F (54.5°C) and pour the next layer (B). Repeat these steps to create as many layers as you want in the soap. Add a final layer of white soap, if desired.

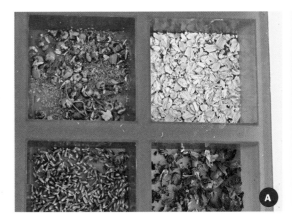

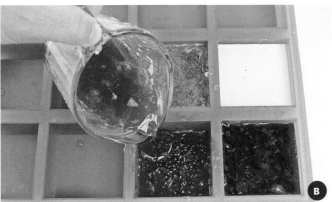

Embedding Shreds and Chunks

Previously made soap can be embedded into new bars of soap. Melt-and-pour soap's transparency and quick hardening allow for a wide range of effects.

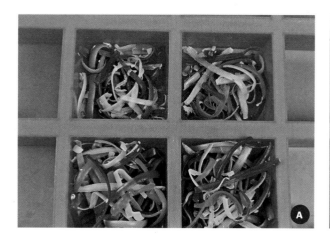

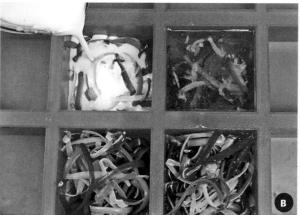

Embedding Simple Shreds of Soap

1 Shred some previously colored soap.

2 Layer or arrange the shredded soap into the mold cavities—as just a top layer or fill the whole mold (A).

3 Melt the soap base for the overpour and add fragrance oil or color as desired. Let the soap base cool to about 130°F (54.5°C).

4 Lightly spray the shreds with rubbing alcohol.

5 Gently pour the melted soap base over the shreds in a zigzag motion to ensure the soap base surrounds all the shreds (B).

Layered Flower with Shreds

1 Shred some green melt-and-pour soap.

2 Melt 1 ounce (28 g) clear soap base (it will take just a few seconds) and stir in a bit of orange mica.

3 Pipe the melted orange soap into the center of the flower mold (A). Let this cool.

4 Melt about 4 ounces (112 g) clear soap base for the flower petals. Stir in about ⅛ teaspoon yellow mica, or any color you prefer.

5 Lightly spray the first (orange) layer with rubbing alcohol.

6 When the yellow soap cools to about 130°F (54.5°C), pour that in and let that layer cool and harden (B).

7 Place the green shreds into the mold cavity (C).

8 Melt enough clear or white soap base to fill the remaining molds. Let the soap base cool to about 130°F (54.5°C).

Should Fragrance Be Added to the Shreds?

It's not a problem if the shreds have fragrance in them, but it's not required. If the shreds are intended to be used as shreds, they can be left unscented and the overpour can be scented. If they are part of another scented soap project, keep that in mind when you choose a scent for the overpour.

9 Lightly spray the shreds with rubbing alcohol.

10 Gently pour the clear or white melted soap over the shreds in a zigzag motion to ensure the soap base surrounds all the shreds (D).

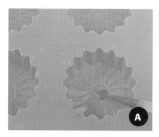 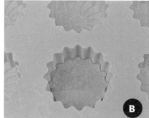 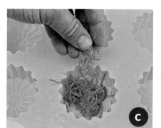 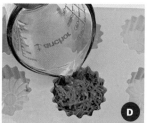

Layered Flower with Shreds.

Additional Techniques for Embedding Shreds and Chunks

These soaps all use chunks and shreds made from the layered melt-and-pour project on page 47 (pictured in the second row in photo on page 39), but these effects can be created with any type of colored soap shreds or chunks.

Confetti Chunks

1. With a cheese grater or mandoline slicer, cut along the bar's edge to make soap curls.

2. Chop the curls in a variety of angles and sizes.

3. Fill the mold cavity with the chopped curls.

4. Lightly spray the curls with rubbing alcohol.

5. When the melted soap base cools to about 130°F (54.5°C), gently pour it into the mold.

Plaid Stripes

1. Slice long, thin chunks along the wide side of a bar.

2. Pour a thin (0.25 inch or 6 mm) layer of clear melted (130°F or 54.5°C) soap.

3. Layer the long chunks into the mold horizontally, all in the same direction. Let that layer cool. Lightly spray the first layer with rubbing alcohol. Pour a second layer of melted soap into the mold.

4. Layer shorter chunks vertically into the mold. Let that layer cool.

5. Repeat the horizontal and vertical layers to create as many layers as needed to fill the mold.

Striped Chunks

1. Chop a bar of soap into chunks of assorted sizes.

2. Fill the mold cavity with the chunks.

3. Lightly spray the chunks with rubbing alcohol.

4. When the melted soap base cools to about 130°F (54.5°C), gently pour it over the chunks.

Millefiori Curls

This technique uses soap curls to suggest a millefiori effect.

1. With a cheese grater or mandoline slicer, cut along the bar's edge to make soap curls. Be careful to keep the curls at their full length. Set aside any that break in half. Pour a thin (0.25 inch or 6 mm) layer of melted clear soap base into the mold.

2. Arrange the curls in the mold standing up, filling as much space as possible with curls.

3. Lightly spray the curls with rubbing alcohol.

4. Pour another layer of clear soap into the mold.

5. Fill the rest of the mold with clear or white soap as a backdrop.

STAINED-GLASS EMBEDDED SOAPS

Light flowing through colored, transparent soap can create beautiful and unexpected effects. These soaps use liquid dyes for maximum transparency and so will be prone to color bleed, however the mica-colored gray soap "cames" or "canes" between the clear pieces of soap "glass" will buffer the color bleed.

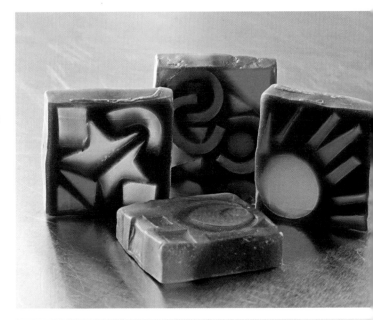

1 Cut and create a variety of shapes from transparent, colored clear soap—either from whole bars or scraps of other bars (A).

2 Weigh the shapes. Arrange them in a slab mold or (as shown here) in individual cavity molds (B). (These six soaps use 10 ounces [283.5 g] of embed shapes.)

3 Calculate the amount of overpour you need by subtracting the weight of the embeds (here, 10 ounces or 283.5 g) from the total weight of the final soaps being made (in this case, 24 ounces or 680 g). Melt the overpour amount needed (in this case, 14 ounces or 396.5 g) clear soap base. Stir in ¼ teaspoon silver or gray mica.

4 When the gray soap cools to about 130°F (54.5°C), lightly spray the embeds with rubbing alcohol and pour the gray soap over the embeds, being careful not to disturb the pieces as much as possible (C).

5 As some gray overpour will inevitably seep under the embeds and be poured over the embeds, you'll need to plane the soap on a soap planer or mandoline slicer to get a clean face on the soap to reveal the embeds. It will seem like a waste of soap, but the final effect is worth it.

Makes 6 soaps

How Much Overpour Should I Prepare?

To calculate how much soap to melt for the overpour:

1 Note the mold size and weight of the final soap.

2 Weigh the shreds being added to the soap.

3 Subtract the weight of the shreds from the final soap weight to determine the amount of overpour to prepare.

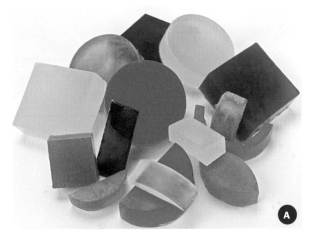

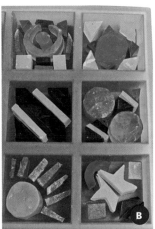

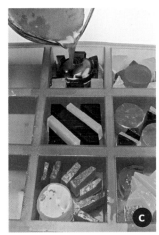

More Layered and Embedded Projects

The truly marvelous thing about melt-and-pour soap is its ability to be layered, embedded, colored, and molded into incredible designs. Here are a few examples.

LAYERED STAR SOAPS

1 Using the basic technique (see page 43), make four small star soap embeds with white soap base in a soap or chocolate mold.

2 Melt about 4 ounces (112 g) clear soap base.

3 Stir in ¼ teaspoon cosmetic glitter. Keep stirring gently until the soap cools to about 120°F (49°C).

4 Pour 0.5 inch (1 cm) clear soap into the star molds (A).

5 Gently place the white star embeds into the mold cavities just deep enough for the star to be even with the melted soap. Position the embeds with a chopstick, if needed. Let this layer cool and harden (B).

6 Melt 12 ounces (336 g) clear soap base.

7 Add about ⅛ teaspoon (0.6 ml) blue mica to the melted soap—just enough to color it lightly.

8 Lightly spray the first layer with rubbing alcohol. Pour about 0.25 inch (6 mm) blue soap into each mold cavity. Let this layer cool enough to form a skin. It does not need to harden completely (C).

9 Stir another bit of blue mica into the remaining soap. Reheat to about 130°F (54.5°C), if necessary.

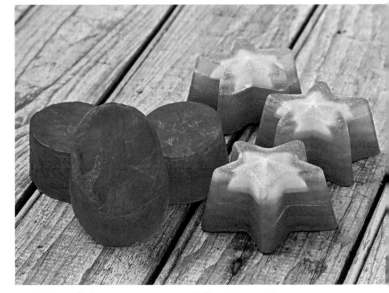

Luffa Soaps (left, see recipe on page 54) and Layered Star Soaps (right).

10 Spray the cooled second layer again with rubbing alcohol. Pour another layer of the (now a bit darker) melted blue soap.

11 Repeat the blue layers, adding a bit more colorant, and pouring layers until the mold cavities are full.

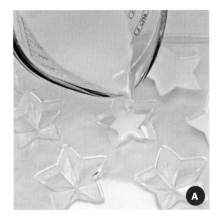

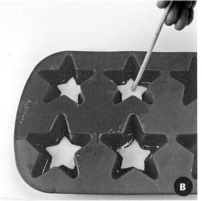

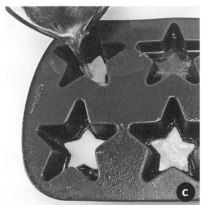

LUFFA SOAPS

Luffa (also spelled loofah) sponges come from the fibrous centers of a plant in the cucumber family. The luffa can be ground and added to soap as a natural exfoliant, or slices of sponge can be placed in individual soap molds.

1 Place a slice of luffa into each mold cavity. For exfoliation throughout the soap, make the slice as deep as the mold cavity. For a scrubby side and a smooth side, make the slice half as deep as the cavity, as shown (A).

2 For these three (3 ounces or 85 g) bars, melt 9 ounces (255 g) clear soap base and stir in 0.25 ounce (7 g) fragrance oil and colorant of choice.

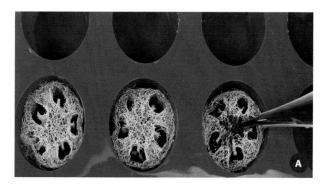

3 Pour the melted soap over the luffa slices. They tend to float to the top of the mold. Use a chopstick to push them back to the bottom of the mold so the luffa will be on the soap's top. (See photo on page 53, top left, for the finished soap.)

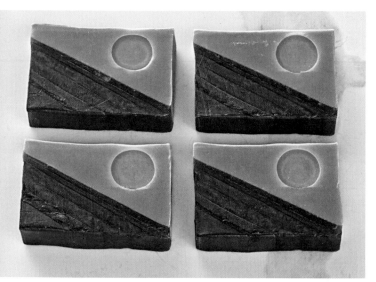

DESERT SUN

One wonderful aspect of melt-and-pour soap making is the ability to create and sculpt designs. This recipe is based on a loaf mold that holds 44 ounces (1.25 kg) of soap. Progressively less mica is used in the brown layers to produce an ombré effect.

1 Make the sun embed in a small, round soap mold or with a length of PVC pipe. Melt about 4 ounces (113 g) clear soap base and add ¼ teaspoon orange mica (A). Set aside to cool. You will likely need to freeze the soap for about 20 minutes to get it to slide out of the mold.

2 Tilt the loaf mold at approximately a 45-degree angle so the "horizon" stretches from about 0.5 inch (1 cm) above the bottom corner to 0.5 inch (1 cm) below the mold's top corner.

3 Melt 3 ounces (85 g) clear melt-and-pour soap. Stir in ½ teaspoon brown mica and 0.1 ounce (3 g) fragrance. Pour this into the bottom of the tilted mold. Let this layer cool (B).

4 Melt 3 more ounces (85 g) clear soap base. Stir in a bit less than ½ teaspoon brown mica and 0.1 ounce (3 g) fragrance. Spray the first layer with rubbing alcohol. Pour the next layer on top when it has cooled to about 130°F (54.5°C).

5 Repeat the brown layers, for a total of six, adding progressively less and less mica with each layer so the final layer has just enough mica to color the soap lightly (C). Let this last layer cool.

6 Melt 22 ounces (623.7 g) white soap base. Stir in 0.7 ounce (21 g) fragrance and just enough blue mica to create a sky-blue color.

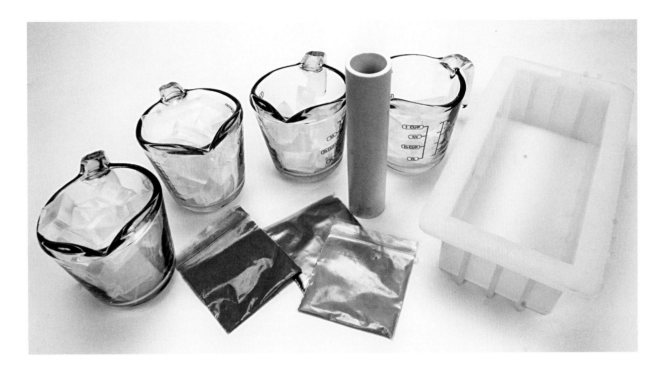

7 Place the mold flat on the table and pour about 10 ounces (283.5 g) melted blue soap into the mold—just enough so the blue soap fills about halfway up the edge of the brown soap (D).

8 Let the blue layer cool just enough so a thick skin forms— enough to hold the weight of the embed—but still a bit warm. Place the sun embed into the mold (E).

9 Reheat the blue soap to 130°F (54.5°C).

10 Spray the blue layer and the orange embed with rubbing alcohol. Pour the remaining blue soap into the mold, being careful not to move the embed (F).

11 Let the soap cool and harden completely.

Makes about 44 ounces (1.25 kg)

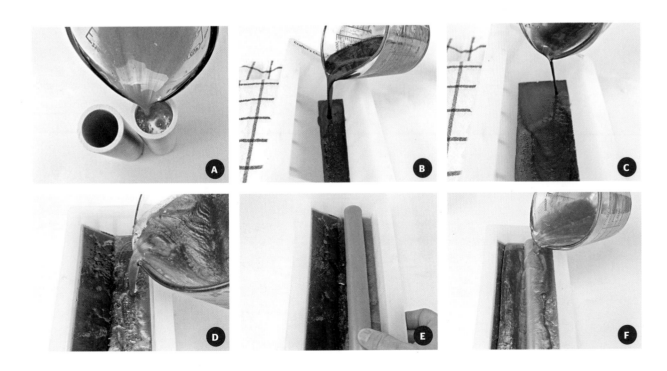

Swirling Melt-and-Pour Soap

Swirl effects can be achieved in a melt-and-pour soap base, but they are a bit more difficult to make. Because the soap base is more fluid when it's hot but thickens quickly, swirls that can be made in slower-moving cold process soaps just aren't possible. However, some marvelous effects can be created with combinations of clear and white bases and multiple layers.

Basic Melt-and-Pour Swirls

The key to melt-and-pour swirls is swirling the soaps at just the right temperature. That "right" temperature will depend on the effect you want.

- For a more fluid, marbled, or variegated effect, swirl the bases together at 130°F to 135°F (54.5°C to 57°C).

- For more defined colors and designs, swirl the soaps together at 120°F to 125°F (49°C to 51.5°C).

- To have one color more defined than the other, pour that color 5°F to 10°F (3°C to 5.5°C) cooler than the first. For example, swirl soap at 120°F to 125°F (49°C to 51.5°C) into soap that is 130° (54.5°C).

Swirling Melt-and-Pour Soap in Slab Mold

Melt-and-pour soap can also be swirled in a slab mold like cold process soap. This recipe uses a 9-inch (23 cm) silicone cake mold to make nine (3-inch or 7.5 cm) square bars of soap.

1 Melt 36 ounces (1 kg) clear melt-and-pour soap base. Stir in 1 ounce (28 g) fragrance oil. Separate the soap base into as many containers as you have colors chosen (A). For this slab swirl, the soap should be at about 135°F (57°C). (This is a great project to keep the measuring cups resting in a slow cooker or pan of warm water to keep the soap melted.)

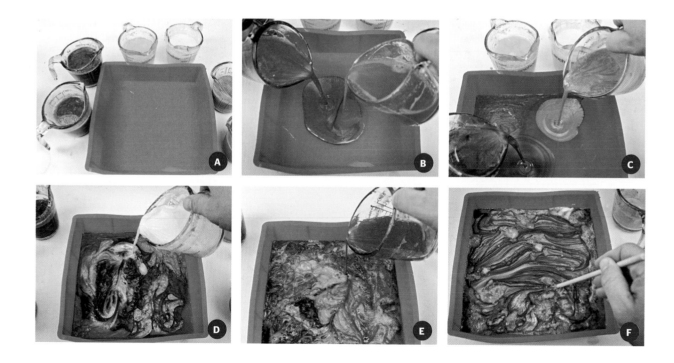

2 Stir mica or other nonbleeding colorant into the individual containers. For six containers with 6 ounces (170 g) of soap each, use about ¼ teaspoon mica in each.

3 Start by pouring two colors simultaneously so they cover about half the mold bottom (B).

4 Pour two more colors simultaneously so the bottom is now mostly covered (C).

5 Layer additional colors in zigzag or circular motions into the melted soap (D).

6 Continue pouring and layering the melted soap until all the soap is poured (E).

7 The pouring motion, alone, creates a swirl effect in the soap. If a more swirled effect is desired, slowly drag a chopstick through the soap, back and forth in an *S* shape, to add additional swirls (F).

Basic Single-Cavity Mold Swirl

1 Melt 12 ounces (340 g) clear soap base and 4 ounces (113 g) white soap base. (A)

2 Add 0.4 ounce (11 g) fragrance oil to the clear base and 0.1 ounce (2.8 g) to the white base.

3 Separate the clear soap into two containers. Stir about ⅛ teaspoon blue mica into one of the containers.

4 Pour about 0.25 inch (6 mm) clear soap into each of four mold cavities (B).

5 Check the temperatures of the three soap bases. Reheat them or let them cool so they are all about 125°F (51.5°C).

6 Simultaneously pour about 0.5 inch (1 cm) blue and clear soaps into the molds (C).

7 From 6 to 8 inches (15 to 20 cm) above the mold, so the white soap penetrates down into the blue and clear mixture, pour about 3 tablespoons (35 g) white soap in a zigzag motion into the molds (D).

8 With a chopstick, give each mold a very light swirl (E).

9 Let the soap set for 2 to 3 minutes. Lightly spray it with rubbing alcohol and repeat the blue/clear pour with the white swirl again to fill the molds.

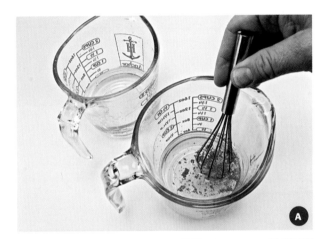
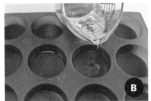
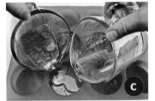
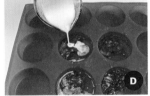
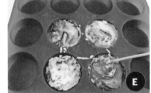

Variations

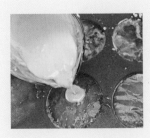

- Use 10 ounces (283.5 g) clear and 6 ounces (170 g) white soap base. Follow the steps listed previously, but use the extra white soap to form the soap's base. This will give it a contrasting background and help the blue stand out more.
- Use any combination of micas and/or clear soap you like.

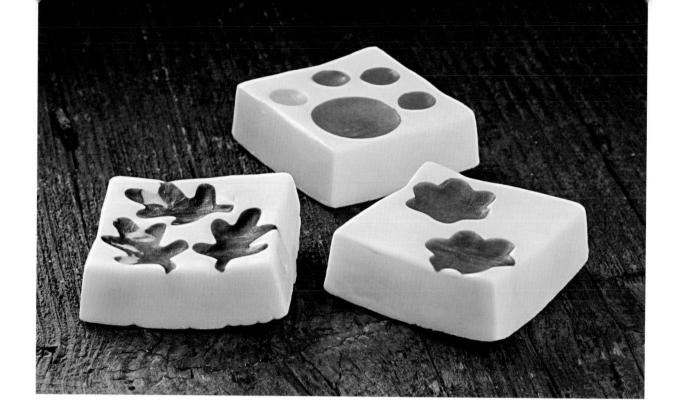

Cookie Cutter Embed Soaps

This recipe uses a bar of swirled soap (see page 56) to create embedded pieces of soap, and plain white soap is used as an overpour around the embeds.

1 Using several bars of premade soap, cut out embeds using small cookie cutters (A). Note the total weight of all the embeds.

2 Arrange the embeds in single-cavity molds (B).

3 Calculate the total weight of the finished soaps and subtract the weight of the embeds. This gives you the amount of soap to melt for the overpour.

4 Melt the appropriate amount of overpour and stir in the fragrance. If the embeds are already scented from their original batches, just calculate enough fragrance for the overpour (about 3 percent by weight). If they are not already scented, use more fragrance in the overpour (4 to 5 percent by weight).

5 For this recipe, we are making six (4-ounce or 113 g) soaps with 10 ounces (283.5 g) of embeds. So, 24 ounces (680 g) of finished soaps minus 10 ounces (283.5 g) of embeds = 14 ounces (396.5 g) of overpour. The embeds are already scented, so about 0.4 ounce (11 g) fragrance oil is added to the overpour.

6 Let the melted overpour soap cool to 125°F to 130°F (51.5°C to 54.5°C).

7 Lightly spray the embeds with rubbing alcohol and gently pour the overpour over the embeds (C). Reposition them with a chopstick if needed.

8 Let the soaps cool and harden.

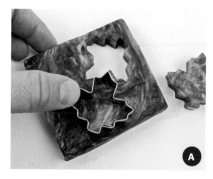
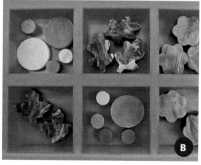
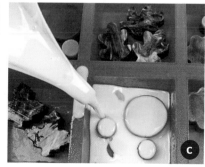

Whipped Melt-and-Pour Soaps

Melt-and-pour soap can be whipped into a light, airy consistency and can be used on its own or for a frosting-like effect or embellishment in other kinds of soap projects.

1 Add 2 tablespoons (30 ml) liquid soap (make sure it is real soap, not dish detergent) to 4 ounces (113 g) white melt-and-pour soap base (A).

2 Melt the mixture to about 150°F (65.5°C).

3 In a large measuring cup, slowly whip the melted soap with an electric mixer.

4 The soap will first foam and bubble up considerably. (That's the reason to use a large measuring cup.) Keep whipping. It will settle down and thicken. The whipping isn't causing the thickening. The soap thickens as it cools (B).

5 Keep whipping the soap until it reaches your desired consistency for use in your project. If it gets too thick, reheat it for several seconds and stir thoroughly (C).

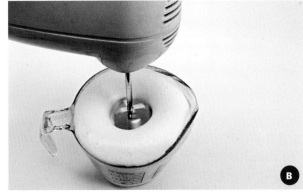

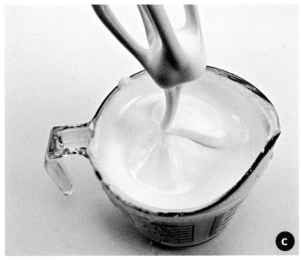

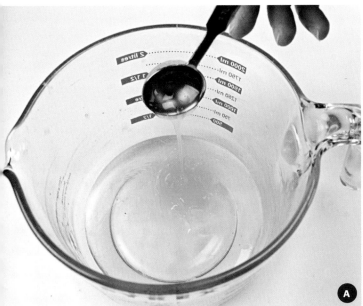

Some Whipped-Soap Project Ideas

1 Put the whipped soap into a cookie press or piping bag to create individual soap "cookies."

2 Pour the whipped soap into ice cube trays or brownie molds for soap "marshmallows."

3 Top a standard melt-and-pour "cupcake" with soap "frosting."

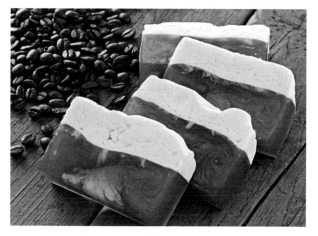

COFFEE MELT-AND-POUR SOAP

This recipe combines a coffee-colored clear base swirled with white soap as "cream" and topped with a white whipped-soap topping. It uses a 44-ounce (1.25 kg) loaf mold.

1 Melt 24 ounces (680 g) clear soap base and 6 ounces (170 g) white soap base.

2 Stir 0.8 ounce (22.6 g) fragrance oil into the clear base and 0.2 ounce (5.6 g) into the white base. (Be careful about using vanilla-based fragrances. Although the "coffee" section can shift a bit brown, you don't want the cream to turn brown.)

3 Stir about ¼ teaspoon coffee-colored mica into the clear base—just enough to give the soap a brown yet transparent color.

4 To begin pouring, have the clear soap base at 130°F (54.5°C) and the white base at 120°F (49°C).

5 Pour the brown soap into the loaf mold (A).

6 From 3 inches (7.5 cm) away, drizzle the white soap into the brown soap in a zigzag motion, like drizzling cream into coffee (B). If the white soap sinks too far to the bottom, let both soaps cool a bit more. You want the cream swirls to be suspended in the coffee base.

7 Let the coffee and cream base cool enough to form a firm skin on top.

8 Melt 4 ounces (113 g) white soap and 2 tablespoons (30 ml) liquid soap together.

9 Whip the soaps together until creamy and light peaks form (C).

10 Pour the whipped soap over the top of the coffee and cream base (D).

11 If desired, sculpt the whipped top as it cools (E).

Makes 8 (1-inch or 2.5 cm) bars

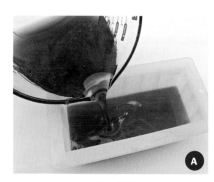

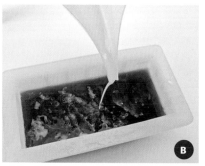

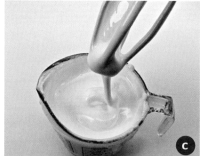

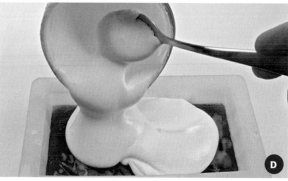

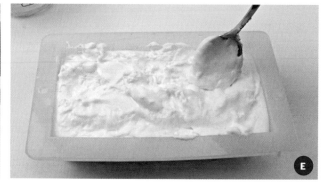

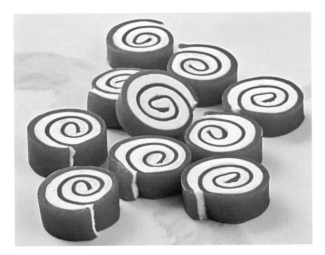

JELLY ROLL MELT-AND-POUR SOAP

1 Melt 6 ounces (170 g) clear soap base. Stir in 3 tablespoons (45 ml) liquid glycerin and 0.20 ounce (5.6 g) fragrance oil. (The added glycerin makes the soap pliable even after it cools.)

2 Stir in 0.25 teaspoon pink mica. Pour the soap into a 9-inch (23 cm) slab mold (A).

3 When the pink layer is cool, melt together 2 ounces (56.5 g) white soap and 1 tablespoon (15 ml) liquid soap.

4 Whip the melted soap until it is light and creamy (B).

5 Lightly spray the first layer with rubbing alcohol. Pour the whipped soap over the pink layer (C). Smooth it so it is even. Let the two layers cool.

6 Gently unmold the soap and lay it on a flat surface.

7 Slowly bend about 0.5 inch (1 cm) of the soap over to begin the roll (D).

8 Continue slowly rolling the soap tightly (E).

9 Drizzle a bit of melted clear soap onto the last edge to glue the roll shut (F).

10 Slice the soap roll into small individual soaps.

Makes 8 (1 ounce or 28 g) slices of jelly roll soap

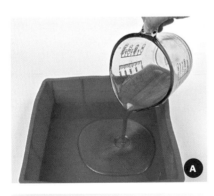
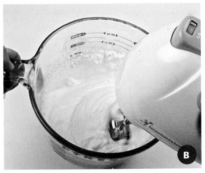
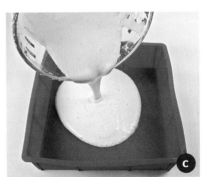
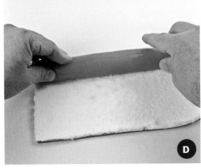
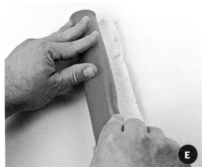
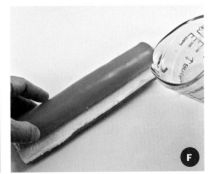

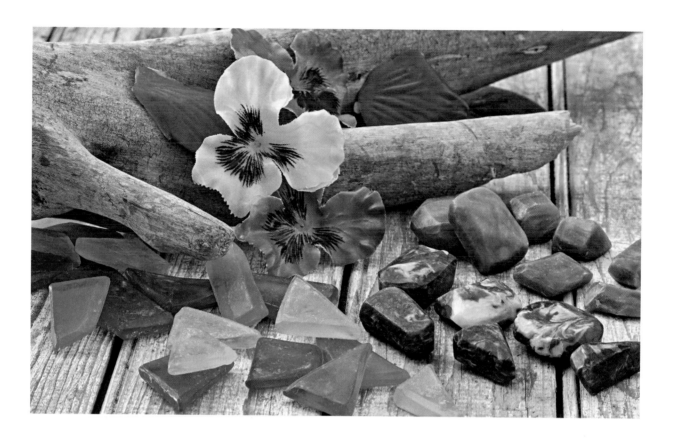

Single-Use and Guest Soaps

Because melt-and-pour soap can be melted in very small batches and made quickly, it is a great soap for seasonal, decorative, and single-use soaps. A bowl of these next to the guest bathroom sink not only makes the room smell lovely, but also delights anyone using them.

GEM STONE AND SEA GLASS SOAPS

The transparent and high-gloss look of melt-and-pour soap can be made to look like gems, glass, or polished stones.

1 Melt 8 ounces (227 g) clear soap base. Stir in 0.25 ounce (7 g) fragrance oil.

2 Separate the melted soap into four portions. Color each portion with a few drops of liquid dye colorant. Unlike layered or swirled projects, we can use dyes for these soaps because we want the soap to be as transparent as possible, and we don't have to worry about color bleed because each soap is just one color.

3 After the colored soaps harden, cut each of them into random shapes (A).

4 With a vegetable peeler, carve the edges and faces of the soaps in a variety of directions and depths (B). Bevel some the edges. Leave some flat. Angle some of the faces. Cut grooves or gouges in others.

5 To keep the soaps looking like gemstones, leave them as carved (C). To give them a more weathered, matte-finish look like sea glass, lightly rub a bit of kaolin, bentonite clay, or cornstarch into the soap pieces.

Yield: Varies

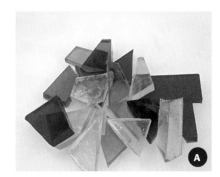

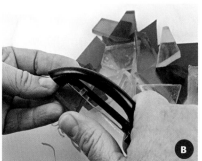

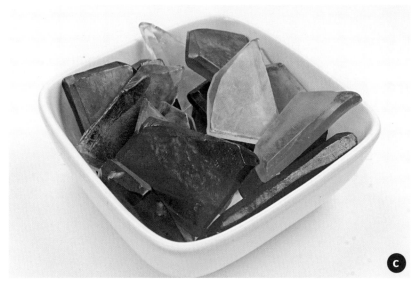

SOAP STONES

Soaps that look like stones, geodes, or crystals can be crafted from melt-and-pour soap as well as by using clays and micas (especially metallic tones) in either swirled, chunk, or shred-based soaps.

1 Using the same technique as the Gem Stone and Sea Glass Soaps (opposite), take a bar of melt-and-pour soap swirled with mica (see page 56), or any bar of multicolored, variegated soap, and carve stones out of it. Because the bar of soap is thicker, you'll be able to carve rounder stones. Larger stones or crystals can be constructed out of larger chunks of clear, transparent soap mixed with gemstone-colored micas. "Veins" of metallic mica can be created by brushing mica onto the chunks and then pouring melted soap over the chunks.

2 When you've completed your "stones," rub them with a paper towel or soft cloth to smooth any edges. You can also polish them further by rubbing them under running water. (See photo opposite, far right, for the finished soaps.)

Yield: Varies

DIPPED SOAP PETALS

This recipe infuses artificial flower petals with clear soap to create beautiful single-use soaps. Choose petals from a favorite flower or for a particular season or occasion.

1 Separate a dozen or so artificial flower petals from their stems (A). Before you use them, make sure they are color safe by running one under hot water and rubbing it with a little dish soap.

2 Melt about 6 ounces (170 g) clear soap base. Stir in about 0.25 ounce (7 g) fragrance oil. This dipping soap works best when it is warm and fluid—about 140°F to 150°F (60°C to 65.5°C).

3 Gently dip each flower petal into the soap base, letting them soak in the melted soap for a few seconds. Remove and let the excess drip off (B).

4 Place the petals on a piece of waxed paper to harden (C).

5 Place the petals in a bowl next to the sink for hand washing.

Makes 12 soap petals

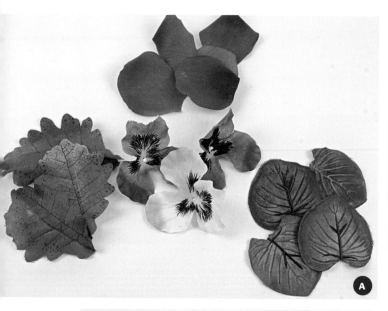

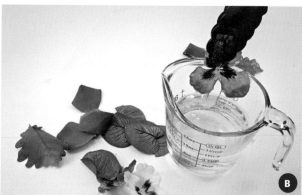

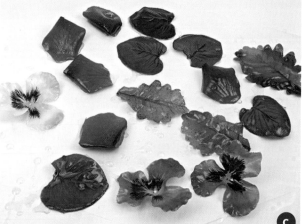

Variations

Instead of flower petals, any small, soft piece of fabric or felt can be used. Seasonal patterns, monogramed squares, or even felt snowflakes and ornaments can be used.

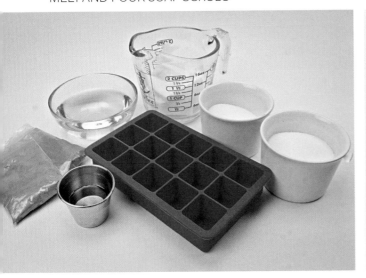

Ingredients and equipment for melt-and-pour sugar scrubs.

INGREDIENTS

- 3 ounces (85 g) white melt-and-pour soap base
- 2.5 ounces (71 g) light oil, such as almond, sunflower, or grape seed
- 0.5 ounce (14 g) liquid glycerin
- Mica or liquid colorant (optional)
- 0.2 ounce (5.6 g) fragrance oil or essential oil (optional)
- 9 ounces (255 g) granulated salt or sugar

Yield: Varies

Sugar and salt scrubs are a popular method of exfoliating and moisturizing your skin. Generally, they are formulations of oil, fragrance, and either sugar or salt packaged in plastic jars. Each time you want to use the scrub, just scoop out a bit, rub it into your skin, and rinse it off.

These scrubs are made with melt-and-pour soap as a base that makes them more convenient and neater to use. Just grab one cube and scrub. The soap in the mixture helps the oil rinse off your skin (and down the drain) more cleanly, too.

1 Melt the soap base in the microwave. Stir in the light oil, fragrance oil, and colorant (if using) (A).

2 If necessary, reheat the oil and soap mixture, very briefly, to about 140°F (60°C).

3 Stir the salt or sugar into the soap and oil mixture.

4 The mixture will thicken quickly as you stir. Reheat the mixture again, very briefly, to about 140°F (60°C).

5 Pour the mixture into an ice cube tray, mini-muffin pan, or any other small-cavity mold, where each cube will weigh about 1.5 ounces (42.5 g) (B).

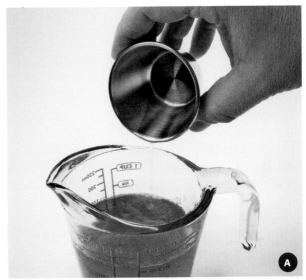

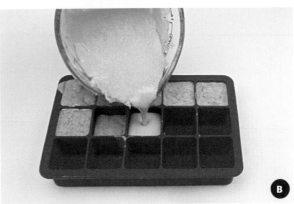

Melt-and-Pour Soap: Tips and Troubleshooting

While melt-and-pour soap may seem most suited for beginners, there are practically limitless design possibilities. Whether beginner or advanced, here are some tips to make the best soaps possible.

Tips for Melt-and-Pour Soaps

1   Use a quality soap base. There are many types of melt-and-pour soap bases available. Soap suppliers generally sell the best ones.

2   Watch the soap temperature carefully. The range of temperatures where the soap is too cool or too hot is narrow. Most bases will be most mixable and pourable between 130°F and 140°F (54.5°C to 60° C).

3   Use scraps as "ice cubes" to cool the soap (A).

4   Don't burn the soap. Once the soap base is heated above 160°F (71°C), it will start to boil and burn. Burned soap has a gloppy, leathery texture when melted (B).

5   Melting and pouring temperatures can vary between soap base brands. Use the temperatures recommended here as starting points and adjust for the soap base you are using.

6   While soap can be reheated/remelted, it will lose water each time you heat it. Covering the container with plastic wrap can help minimize water loss.

7   For more intricate or complex designs, melt the soap in small containers and keep them warm in a pan or slow cooker full of warm water (C). This gives you more time to work before the soap begins to cool and harden.

8   While a bit of extra oil can be a good thing in cold process soap, with melt-and-pour soap it tends to make the soap softer and stickier and reduces the lather as well. If you want a luxury ingredient, such as shea butter or goat's milk, in your soap, it's best to purchase a base with it already formulated into the recipe.

9   When trying to keep botanicals or other items suspended in soaps, moving the mold to the refrigerator immediately after pouring can help cool and harden the soaps more quickly.

10   Always use the same brand of soap base in layered or swirled soaps. Different brands of soap contain slightly different ingredients in them and harden and dry at different rates. This can cause the layers to be more prone to separating.

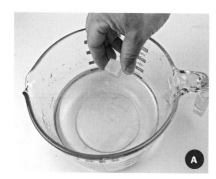
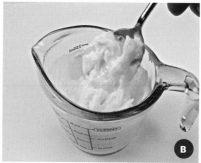
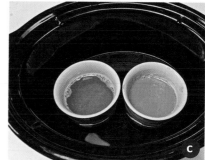

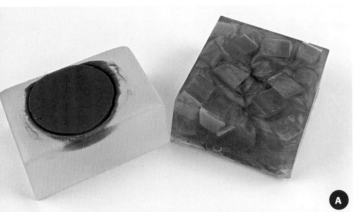

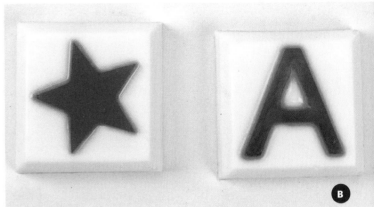

Troubleshooting Melt-and-Pour Soaps

1   **The additives sank to the bottom of the mold.** The soap base was too warm when poured. Let the soap cool (and thicken) before pouring it into the mold, or use a suspension base.

2   **The soap is stuck in the mold.** Some soap molds, especially single-cavity molds, can be difficult to unmold. Adding liquid or oil additives can also make the soap stickier. Make sure the soap is completely cool. Slowly and gently try to push the soap out, bit by bit. If it still resists, refrigerate the soap for 30 minutes and try again.

3   **The layers separated.** To help soap layers adhere, pour the second layer while the first layer is cooled enough to have formed a skin on top, but is still a bit warm. Also, spritz a bit of rubbing alcohol on the first layer before you pour the second.

4   **The embed or second layer melted the first layer.** The second, or overpour, layer was too hot (A). While you can pour the first layer at 140°F to 150°F (60°C to 65.5°C), second layers and overpours should be between 125°F and 135°F (51.5°C and 57°C).

5   **The botanicals I added turned moldy.** Fresh or puréed additives can begin to mold in the soap. Use only fully dried botanicals in soaps.

6   **The soap is thick and leathery in the measuring cup.** It's likely the soap is old, or has been burned by multiple meltings. While it may not be brown, enough water has evaporated from the soap base to cause this. Work with it as you can, or discard it.

7   **My soap looks like it is sweating.** Melt-and-pour soap contains a lot of glycerin, which is a humectant (attracts water). The soap is attracting moisture from the air. After it cools, wrap the soap in plastic wrap. Even if this is not your final packaging, it will help keep the soap from sweating and can be taken off when you are ready to package, sell, or use the soap.

8   **The colored embeds have a foggy, colored halo around them.** You are probably seeing "color bleed," which happens in soap, especially melt-and-pour soaps, when you use water-soluble liquid dyes (B). Use nonbleeding colors, such as micas or oxides, and the colors won't bleed.

Making Cold Process Soap

Though the process has been around for thousands of years, it was just in the 1970s that handmade natural soap making really started growing as a craft, hobby, and business. The cold process method of soap making allows crafters to create anything from simple, basic soaps to sumptuous, elegant, designs. The basics are all the same—combine sodium hydroxide with water to make a lye solution, and mix it with some oils. When the soap maker's creativity adds color, scent, and other additives, the raw soap batter is transformed from something everyday into a beautiful, yet practical, addition to your daily life.

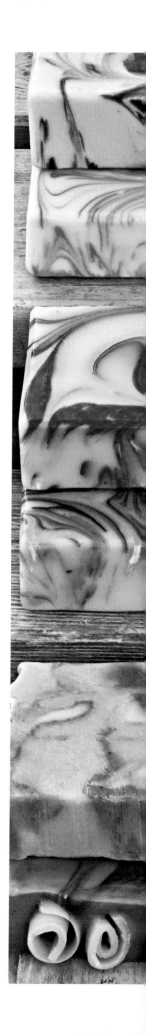

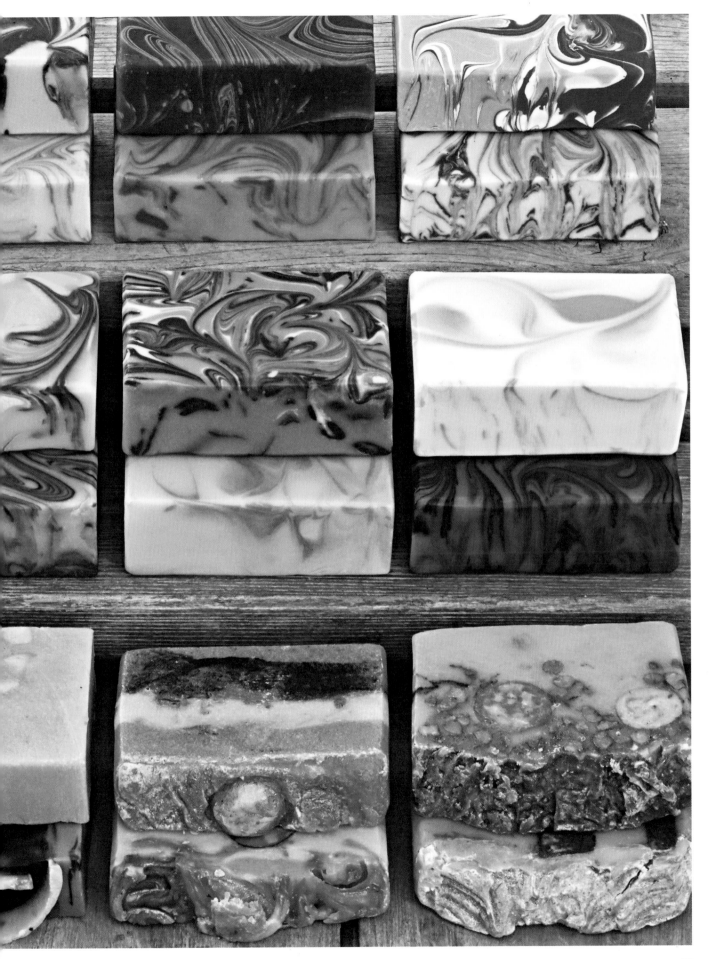

The Basic Components of Cold Process Soap

Soap, at its most basic, is a simple creation that results from a basic chemical reaction. Fats (animal or vegetable oils) are broken apart by an alkali (sodium hydroxide or potassium hydroxide) and recombined into soap and glycerin.

oils + lye = soap + glycerin

But to leave it there would be like stopping after saying that all bread is made with flour and water. While true, it is in the variety and customization of ingredients, additives, and cooking processes that soap is transformed from a blob of white stuff into a wonderful, handcrafted creation.

Soap Ingredients

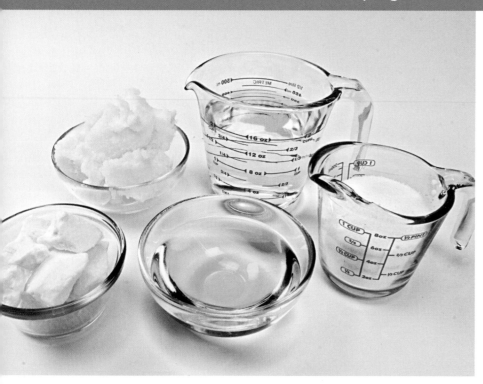

bread, each type of fatty acid gives different qualities to soap.

Lye

The alkali used to break down the oils and transform them into soap is *sodium hydroxide* (for solid bar soap) or *potassium hydroxide* (for liquid soap.) While lye used to be made by leaching rainwater through wood ashes, it is now commercially made.

Water

Water serves as the matchmaker between the oils and the lye. Dissolving the lye in water (or other liquid) is necessary for the chemical reaction to move quickly and smoothly.

Oils

The animal and vegetable oils in soap (just like the oils or fats in food) are made up of triglycerides, which get their name from the three fatty acids joined together by a glycerol molecule. The exact type or combination of fatty acids is different in each oil and, just like different types of flour make different types of

Do I Have to Use Distilled Water?

Many soap makers ask (and most books recommend) that you use distilled water in your soap recipes. Using distilled water is indeed great for soap, especially for beginners, because there are no impurities (such as dissolved metals or minerals) and it is very consistent batch to batch. Some studies have linked impurities in tap water to soap developing spots of rancidity (called "dreaded orange spots" or DOS), but many soap makers around the world use tap water regularly in their soap recipes with no problem at all.

Additional Soap Ingredients

Scent

Natural essential oils or synthetic fragrance oils can be used to scent your soaps. Make sure that whatever scent oils you use are "skin safe"—approved for use in soap.

Color

A wide variety of natural and synthetic colorants is available to give aesthetic appeal to your soap—from subtle to vibrant, simple to wildly complex.

Everything Else

Additional additives are often added to soaps to create even further customization. Exfoliants, liquids other than water, plants and other botanicals, or ingredients included to give special qualities to the soap (such as goat's milk or aloe vera). Some, such as flower petals, may just be aesthetic, others, such as ground oatmeal or goat's milk, affect how the soap works or affects your skin, and others, such as honey or salt, affect the soap's lather or hardness.

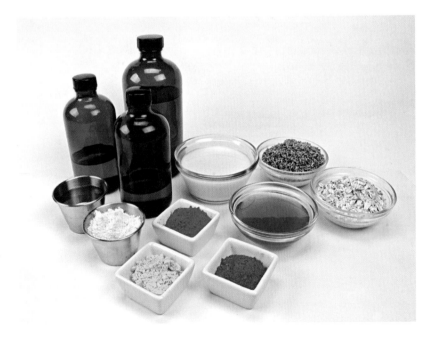

Creating a Cold Process Soap Recipe

Think about the last bar of soap you used. Was the bar hard and dense or light and pliable? Was the lather fluffy with big bubbles or did it have a low, creamy, luxurious lather? Did it leave your skin feeling gently cleansed and moisturized or squeaky clean?

These are all characteristics determined by the oils in a soap recipe. Some oils make a bar that is hard, dense, and long lasting. Other oils contribute to a bubbly, fluffy, high lather. These same oils are also quite cleansing—so much so that too much of them in a bar can be drying to the skin. Other oils give a low, creamier lather, but are moisturizing to the skin.

Creating your own custom soap recipe is one of the great challenges and rewards of making your own soap, and while there are dozens of oils and seemingly limitless variations, soap making oils can be categorized in four ways:

4 WAYS TO CATEGORIZE SOAP MAKING OILS	
Hard	Bubbly
Creamy	Conditioning

Each oil commonly used in soap making has **at least two** of these characteristics:

SOAP MAKING OIL CHARACTERISTISTICS	
Hard and Creamy	Hard and Bubbly
Creamy and Conditioning	Creamy and Bubbly
Hard and Creamy and Conditioning	

Soap can be made using just one oil, but balancing several types of oils in your recipes gives you the best bar of soap and, more importantly, a bar of soap that has exactly the characteristics you love.

The Triumvirate of Oils

1 **Palm oil:** a hard and creamy oil, is one of the most widely used oils in a range of applications including soap making. It makes a hard, long-lasting bar with a low, creamy lather. Due to farming methods and environmental concerns, it has come under quite a bit of scrutiny over the past few years, and many soap makers have chosen to either eliminate it from their recipes or purchase only sustainable palm oil. Substitutes would include animal fats, such as tallow or lard, or nut butters such as cocoa and shea.

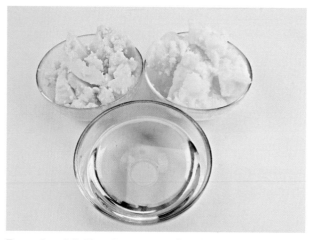

Top: palm oil (left) and coconut oil (right). Bottom: olive oil.

What Kind of Olive Oil Do I Need to Buy?

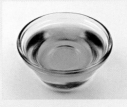

Pomace olive oil.

You'll likely see a few types of olive oil at your grocery store or soap supplier. Any can make great soap, but they have subtle differences, each stemming from where in the oil-extracting process they come from, but not enough to affect the final soap. As long as your oil is fresh and you purchase it from a reliable source (there is growing worldwide concern about adulterated olive oil), use the brand and type that is most available and economical.

1   Extra-virgin or virgin olive oil comes from the first mechanical pressing of the olives and produces the lightest, purest oil.

2   Refined or grade A olive oil comes from the second pressing of the olives and may be partially refined.

3   Pomace olive oil comes from the last bits of olive paste after the virgin and grade A have been pressed out. The last drops of oil are extracted from the skins, pits, and remaining flesh of the olives and, while it doesn't come through in the soap, has a much greener color than the others. Because it doesn't have the flavor the others have, it is mostly relegated to soap and other commercial uses, but it still has the same fatty acid makeup so is just fine to use in soap with one caveat: Pomace oil can contain a lot of unsaponifiables (components of the oil not converted into soap by the lye), so it can tend to speed trace.

2   **Coconut oil:** a hard and bubbly oil that gives a tremendously bubbly lather to soap and makes a super-hard white bar of soap. Coconut oil has a bit of a bad reputation for being drying to your skin. This is because it cleans so well—it is, indeed, cleansing the oils right off your skin. Most soap makers won't use much more than about 30 percent coconut oil in their recipes. Higher amounts can be used if the superfat percentage is increased. The only widely available substitute is palm kernel oil.

3   **Olive oil:** a hard, creamy, *and* conditioning oil, that is great to include in your soap recipes—from 1 to 100 percent. One hundred percent olive oil soap, called Castile soap, is very hard, with a gentle, mild, moisturizing lather. The lather has hardly any bubbles, but is rather thick and almost slimy. Olive oil is more easily substituted for other liquid oils, and its low cost, ready availability, and wonderful results make it widely used in soap making.

Soap Made with Crisco?

Originally formulated in 1911 with hydrogenated cottonseed oil, the recipe for Crisco shortening has changed over the years to include soybean and palm oils as well. It makes good soap, especially if balanced with other oils, but be sure your lye calculator is calibrated for the new formulation. Other shortenings can be used for soap, as well, but it is impossible to calculate the lye amount exactly without knowing the ingredients. So it's best to keep the shortening for frying and single oils for soap making.

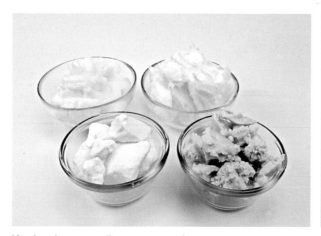
Hard and creamy oils.

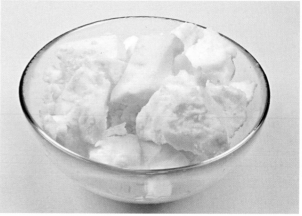
Palm kernel oil, a hard and bubbly oil.

Hard and Creamy

The hard and creamy oils are solid at room temperature and contain mostly palmitic, stearic, and oleic fatty acids. They make a hard, white bar of soap that is long lasting in the shower.

Beef Tallow

Beef tallow is the rendered fat from cows. The density of the fat depends on where in the cow the fat comes from. The fat that surrounds the kidneys, often called suet or leaf fat, makes the best tallow for soap, although any fat you can get from the butcher can be rendered into tallow for soap. It makes a nice, hard, white bar of soap.

Lard

Lard is the rendered fat from pigs. Like beef fat, the density of the fat depends on where on the animal it comes from. Lard is commonly available in the grocery store and is usually partially hydrogenated to extend its shelf life. Lard has a bit more of the creamy fatty acids and fewer hard fatty acids than palm oil. It is also a very good oil to include if you want to create any complex swirls or designs in the soap, as it is known to slow trace.

Cocoa Butter

Cocoa butter, pressed from the cocoa bean, is the key ingredient in chocolate. Unrefined cocoa butter has a wonderful chocolaty scent. Most soap makers prefer the refined and deodorized type that doesn't retain the scent. It contributes both hardness and conditioning qualities to the soap.

Shea Butter

Shea butter is an oil that is solid at room temperature. It comes from the African karité, or shea, tree. While generally known for its great moisturizing and skin-healing qualities, its fatty acid makeup also contributes hardness to the soap.

What Is a SAP Number?

Each oil you use has a SAP or saponification number. This number represents the amount of lye (either sodium hydroxide [NaOH] or potassium hydroxide [KOH]) needed to fully transform 1 gram (0.035 ounce) of oil into soap. It is sometimes expressed as a range or average of numbers because oils can vary in their fatty acid compositions from batch to batch. This variation is one way that superfatting creates a buffer against having too much lye in your soap.

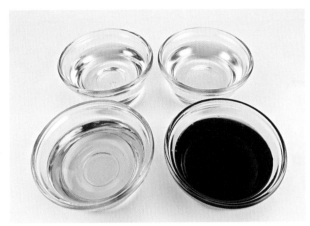

Light creamy and conditioning oils.

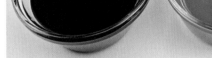

Heavier creamy and conditioning oils.

Hard and Bubbly

These oils contain mostly lauric and myristic fatty acids. In addition to making a very hard white bar of soap, they give fluffy, abundant lather.

Palm Kernel Oil

Though it comes from the same tree as palm oil, palm kernel oil acts more like coconut oil than palm oil in soap—giving a luxurious, bubbly lather. Palm kernel oil is surrounded by the same environmental concerns that palm oil is, however, so coconut is a more popular choice.

Creamy and Conditioning

These oils are liquid at room temperature and come from a wide variety of plants and seeds. They range in color and thickness and contain mostly oleic, linoleic, and linolenic fatty acids.

The Light Liquid Oils

These oils are generally lighter in color and viscosity and are composed of mostly oleic, linoleic, and linolenic fatty acids. While each has unique characteristics (especially if used in other bath and body recipes) in soap, they can be used interchangeably and are a great complement to the hard and bubbly oils. They contribute a creamy lather and make a moisturizing soap. Some of the oils, such as grape seed and hemp oils, have shorter shelf lives and are not as long lasting. Others, such as canola, soybean, and sunflower oils, are more stable as well as being readily available in the grocery store.

Other types include almond, apricot kernel, safflower, and sesame oils.

The Heavier Liquid Oils

Like the light liquid oils, these heavier oils also contain high percentages of oleic, linoleic, and linolenic fatty acids, but they cross over a bit into the hard and creamy category with some palmitic and stearic fatty acid in their composition. Avocado and neem oils also have a lot of unsaponifiables, which are not affected by the lye and come through in the finished soap. Neem oil is known for its antiseptic, antifungal, and other medicinal qualities. Avocado and rice bran oils are sometimes substituted for olive oil. Cottonseed oil is not as widely used anymore, but it used to be the primary ingredient in Crisco shortening.

Creamy and Bubbly
Castor Oil

Castor oil is unique and singular as a soap-making oil as it is the only oil that contains ricinoleic fatty acid. Used at 3 to 8 percent of a soap recipe, it contributes a thick, creamy lather and is mildly conditioning. If used at any higher percentage, it will make a soft, rubbery soap. It also can tend to speed trace, so is best left out of recipes that require a lot of design or swirling.

Making a Lye Solution

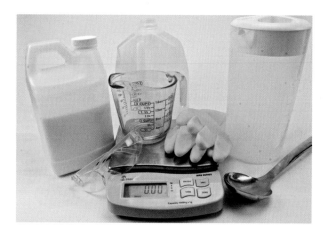

Lye is required to make soap. While there should be no lye remaining when the chemical reaction (saponification) is complete, it is as much a required component of the soap-making process as the oils. That said, *it is also a caustic and corrosive chemical that can cause serious burns if not handled correctly.* Fortunately, with some simple safety gear and procedures, lye solutions for soap making can be made completely safely.

How to Make a Lye Solution

1   Make sure your workspace is clean, organized, well lit, well ventilated, and free from any distractions, such as family or pets. Make sure the other people in your household understand you are working with a chemical that can be dangerous if not handled correctly.

2   In addition to the lye and water, gather all equipment you need to make the lye solution, including

- Soap-making scale
- Lye pitcher: Use plastic (preferred) or a sturdy glass pitcher with at least twice the capacity of the amount of lye solution you are making. This allows you to stir the solution without any chance of spillage. A pitcher with a lid is even safer.
- Measuring cup to weigh the lye: A standard glass measuring cup is fine. As with the pitcher, use one large enough to prevent any spills.
- Stainless steel spoon to stir the solution
- Large pitcher or dish tub in (or near) the sink to put the used utensils in

3   Gather and put on your safety gear, including
- Safety glasses
- Gloves
- Appropriate clothing, such as long sleeves and pants, to cover your arms and legs from any stray droplets

4   Weigh the water.
- Place the lye pitcher onto the scale and zero it out.
- Slowly pour the required amount of water into the pitcher (A).
- If you are adding any additives to your lye solution (such as sugar, salt, colorants, or sodium lactate), stir them in now.
- Set the water pitcher aside.

5   Weigh the lye.
- Place the measuring cup on the scale and zero it out.
- Slowly pour the required amount of lye into the cup (B).
- Set the lye aside.

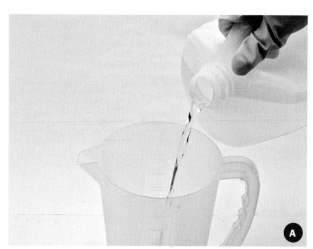

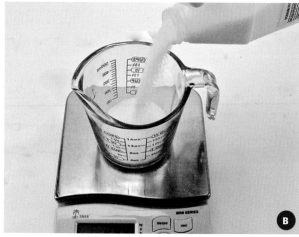

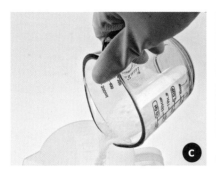
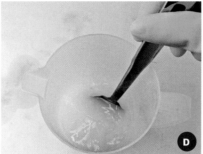
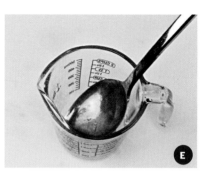

6 Move the scale out of the way and bring back the pitcher of water.

7 Slowly pour the lye into the pitcher of water (C). Often, small bits of lye cling to the bottom of the cup. Gently tap the cup on the counter to dislodge them and pour them into the pitcher.

8 Put the measuring cup used for the lye into the sink, a tub of water, or another safe place. There may still be a few small specks of lye in it.

9 Gently stir the lye solution to dissolve the lye (D). It will immediately begin to heat up to nearly 200°F (93°C) and can give off fumes. Make sure your work area has good ventilation and avoid breathing the fumes while stirring.

10 When the lye is completely dissolved, place the stirring spoon in the same safe place you put the lye measuring cup (E). (Remember, there will be a few droplets of lye solution left on the spoon.)

11 Put the lid on the lye pitcher and set it aside in a safe place to cool.

12 Clean your workspace to ensure no stray lye specks or droplets remain.

Tips for Making Lye Solutions

1 Don't rush. Mistakes and spills are more likely when you're in a hurry.

2 **Always** *add the lye to the water*, not the water to the lye.

3 Make the lye solution near the sink, or have a small dish tub nearby to put the measuring cup and stirring spoon in after you've mixed the solution. Putting them directly into the sink or tub will remind you to handle them properly.

4 Use white vinegar to neutralize any spills or to wipe down your workspace, but *don't use it if you get lye on your skin*. The vinegar reacts with the lye to create even more heat. If you get some lye on you, just flush it very well with water.

5 Safety first. Remember, from the moment the lye is mixed with the water until your soap has finished saponifying, the soap can burn, or at least irritate, your skin or eyes. It's important to keep your safety glasses and gloves on the entire time you are mixing your soap.

Basic Method for Making Cold Process Soap

This basic recipe, which uses four common oils, is a great, reliable recipe for getting started with the cold process method. The steps described and shown are basically the same fundamental steps for all batches of cold process soap. Batches may vary with colorants, additives, and design, but the basic soap-making process remains the same.

INGREDIENTS

- 6.5 ounces (184 g) palm oil
- 6.5 ounces (184 g) coconut oil
- 7.5 ounces (212.6 g) olive oil
- 1 ounce (28 g) castor oil
- 7 ounces (198.5 g) water
- 3.1 ounces (88 g) lye
- 1 ounce (28 g) fragrance oil or essential oil

EQUIPMENT

- 2 lye-safe containers, such as Pyrex, for melting the oils and mixing the soap
- Plastic pitcher for mixing the lye solution
- Small glass container or measuring cup to measure the lye
- Long stainless steel or plastic spoon to mix lye solution
- Stainless steel or plastic whisk
- Rubber spatula
- Immersion or stick blender
- 1 (2 pounds or 907 g) soap mold
- Soap cutter or knife for cutting the finished soap

Makes about 2 pounds (907 g)

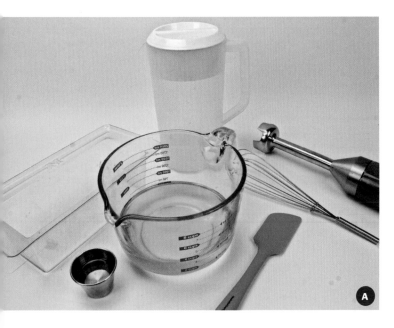

1   Start by assembling all ingredients and equipment, and verifying you have everything you need to make your recipe (A). Put on your goggles and gloves. Make your lye solution (see page 76) and set it aside in a safe place to cool.

2   Weigh the hard oils (the oils that are solid at room temperature) into a glass pitcher (B) and melt them in the microwave. Run the microwave for 1- to 2-minute intervals, stirring in between. When the oils are completely melted, set them aside. Note: To make a larger batch of soap, melt the hard oils in a stainless steel pot on the stovetop.

3   Weigh the liquid oils in a separate container (C). Pour them into the melted hard oils. Note: You can measure and melt all oils at the same time in a single pitcher or pot. However, melting the hard oils first, and adding the room-temperature liquid oils to them, saves some time by helping cool all the oils to the right mixing temperature.

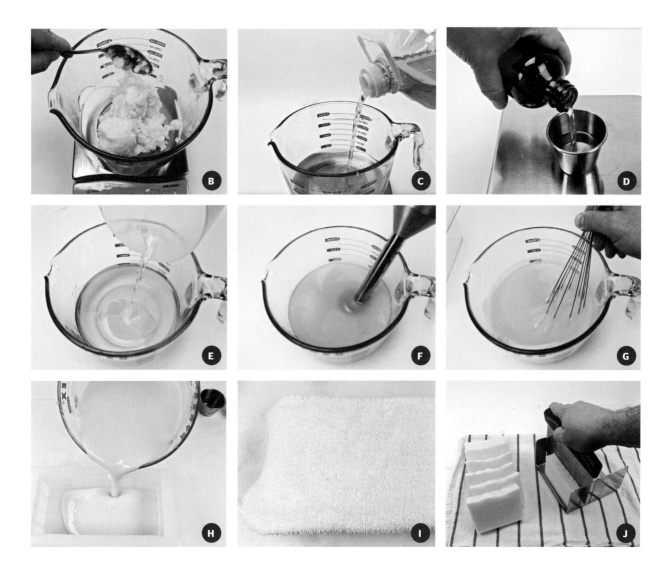

4 While the oils cool, measure the fragrance, essential oil, colorants, and any other additives (D).

5 When the lye solution and oils are both about 100°F to 120°F (38°C to 49°C), it's time to mix them together. Place all the ingredients, tools, additives, and the mold within reach. (Once the oils and lye are mixed together, the chemical reaction starts and the mixture becomes soap quickly!) Slowly and carefully pour the lye solution into the oils and set the lye pitcher aside in a safe place (E). (There will still be some droplets of lye in the pitcher.)

6 Using the immersion blender, mix the oils and lye together using 5- to 10-second bursts. Mix just long enough so the oils and lye are mixed and there are no streaks of oil running through the soap. This first initial emulsification is called *very light trace* (F).

7 Once the oils and lye are fully mixed, it's time to add fragrance, color, or other additives to the soap. Do not use the immersion blender for this; just mix them in with a whisk (G).

8 Slowly pour the soap into the mold (H). Gently tap the mold on the counter to release any air bubbles and help the soap settle into the mold.

9 Cover the soap with a towel (I) and set it aside in a safe, warm place.

10 After 24 to 48 hours, the soap will be firm enough to pop out of the mold and cut. Using a knife or soap cutter, cut the soap into bars (J) and set them in a cool, dry place to cure for 3 to 4 weeks.

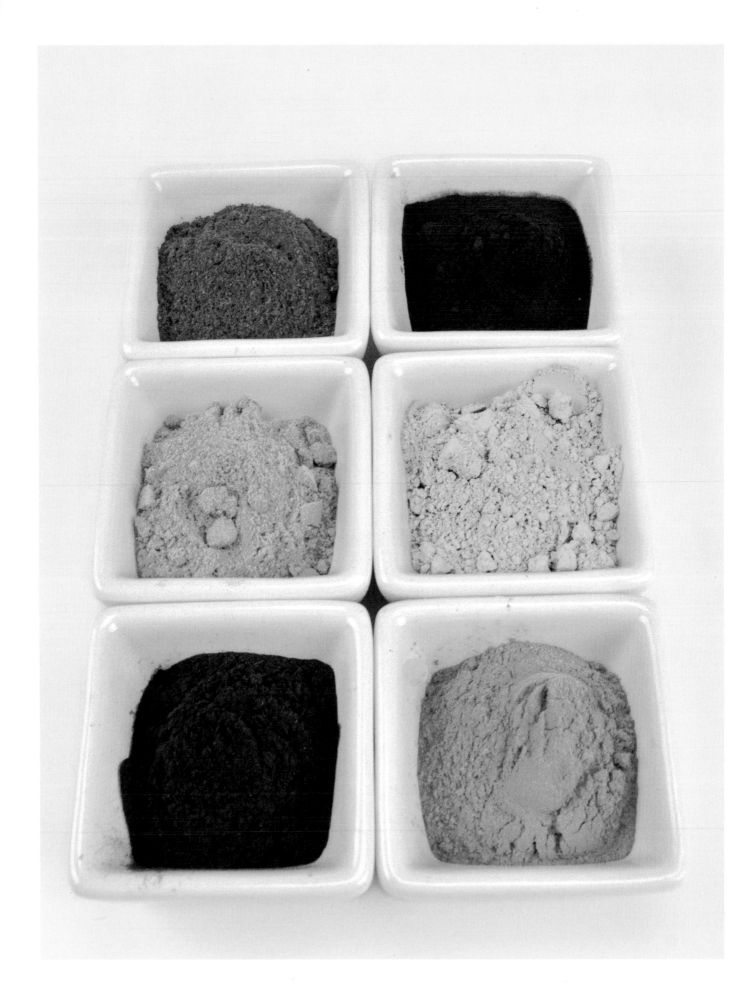

Natural Colors in Cold Process Soap

Micas, oxides, and other synthetic colorants certainly make the most vibrant colors in soap, but natural colorants can be just as interesting and even more varied. Spices, plants, clays, vegetables, and more can be added at various points in the soap-making process.

Some plant materials work best if they are *infused* into one of the base oils, first. Like tea steeping in water, the color infuses into the oil and imparts that color to your soap.

TO MAKE AN INFUSED OIL

To use the infused oil, substitute a portion of the olive oil (25 percent is a good starting point) in your recipe with the infused oil.

INGREDIENTS
- 2 tablespoons (28 g) colorant
- 6 ounces (170 g) olive oil

EQUIPMENT
- Clean glass jar with a lid

Makes about 6 ounces (170 g) infused oil

1 Add the colorant and oil to the jar.

2 Close the jar and label it with the colorant, amount, and date.

3 Shake the jar to mix.

4 Set the jar aside and shake it every day or so for 5 to 6 weeks.

Note: If you don't want to wait 5 to 6 weeks, speed the process along by placing the jar in a slow cooker filled with water. Cover and set the cooker on low heat for 4 to 5 hours. Shake the jars every hour or so.

COLORANTS THAT WORK WELL IN INFUSED OILS			
Annatto: yellow-orange, the color of macaroni and cheese	Alkanet: light to deep purple, depending on the amount used	Paprika: orange-peach	Turmeric: golden amber/brown

Added to the Lye Solution

A few colorants can be added at trace, but they provide a more intense effect if the lye solution is used to draw out the color.

INGREDIENTS

- Lye solution
- 1 to 2 teaspoons (9 to 18.5 g) colorant per 1 pound (454 g) of oils in your recipe

EQUIPMENT

- Cheesecloth or a coffee filter to strain the lye

Yield: Varies

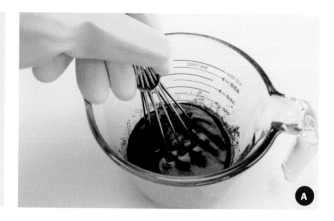

TO MAKE AN INFUSED LYE SOLUTION

1 Make the lye solution for your soap recipe.

2 Carefully wisk in the colorant (A).

3 Set aside the colored lye solution for 2 to 3 hours to steep.

4 Carefully strain the lye solution through layers of cheese-cloth or a coffee filter to strain out the colorant. (Unless you want a speckled effect, in which case don't strain it.)

5 Use the lye solution as you normally would in your soap making.

COLORANTS THAT WORK WELL IN LYE SOLUTION		
Indigo: light to deep blue	Madder root: pinkish-red	Rose clay: deep rose pink

Colorants Added Once the Soap Is Mixed

Many natural colorants can just be added to the soap as it is being made, either to the base oils or at trace. Premix them either with a bit of the soap oils or water, and mix them in at trace as you would any other additive.

COLORANTS THAT WORK WELL ADDED TO THE OILS OR AT TRACE	
Activated charcoal: light gray to deep black	Black walnut hull (ground): speckled brown, also an exfoliant
Calendula flower petals (whole or ground): nice, warm yellow	Carrots (puréed or juiced): muted orange
Cinnamon: reddish tan to brown	Clays (wide variety of colors): white, yellow, pink, brown, green
Cocoa powder: tan to brown	Coffee grounds: dark brown (prone to bleeding, so use already brewed grounds)
Cucumber: pale yellow-green	Kale: deep green
Mint: varied greens (prone to bleeding so steep a tea from the leaves first)	Pumpkin (puréed): orange (can stain some molds)
Rosehips (ground): speckled reddish brown	Sage: muted green
Spinach: deep green	Spirulina: pastel green/blue-green
Tea leaves: varied greens, reds, and browns (prone to bleeding, so use already steeped leaves)	

Making White Soap

What if you want a bright, white bar of soap? There are three ways to make your soap (or a portion of your soap) nice and white:

1 Add titanium dioxide: about 1 teaspoon per 1 pound (454 g) of oils.
2 Adjust your recipe to use a higher percentage of oils that result in whiter soap.

- Beef tallow
- Coconut
- Lard
- Palm kernel

3 Use a colorless fragrance oil or essential oil and none containing vanilla.

Additives for Cold Process Soap Recipes

In addition to color, scent, and exfoliation, there is a variety of other additives for soap recipes.

Additives That Change the Qualities of Soap

Honey: Honey, agave nectar, maple syrup, molasses, and other similar liquid sugars work the same way sugar does in a recipe (see following).

- Add about 1 teaspoon (9 g) per 1 pound (454 g) of oils in the same manner as sugar.

Salt: makes the soap harden more quickly, making unmolding easier.

- Add about 1 teaspoon (9 g) per 1 pound (454 g) of oils to the water *before* adding the lye solution to the water and stir to dissolve fully.

Silk or silk powder: gives soap a shinier appearance and a bit of slip and silkiness.

- Use about 1 teaspoon (9 g) per 1 pound (454 g) of oils, or a small pinch, traditionally the size of a large pea or chickpea. Stir the silk into the hot lye solution; it will take a few minutes to dissolve.

Sodium lactate: a liquid salt derived from fermenting the natural sugars in corn and beets. Like regular salt, it helps the soap harden more quickly and unmold much more easily.

- Use about 1 teaspoon (9 g) per 1 pound (454 g) of oils. Sodium lactate is an amazing additive in hot process soap. Added at the end of the cooking process, it makes the soap significantly more fluid, enhancing the ability to add color, swirl, and mold the soap.

Sugar: helps increase light, bubbly lather.

- Add about 1 teaspoon (9 g) per 1 pound (454 g) of oils to the water *before* adding the lye solution (like with salt). Another option is to subtract a bit of the water, dissolve the sugar in it, and add the sugar-water solution at trace.

Waxes: Soy and beeswax can be added to soap recipes. They provide hardness, primarily, but have also been known to reduce ash on soap.

- Adding more than 3 percent of the total recipe dampens the lather and makes the soap sticky.

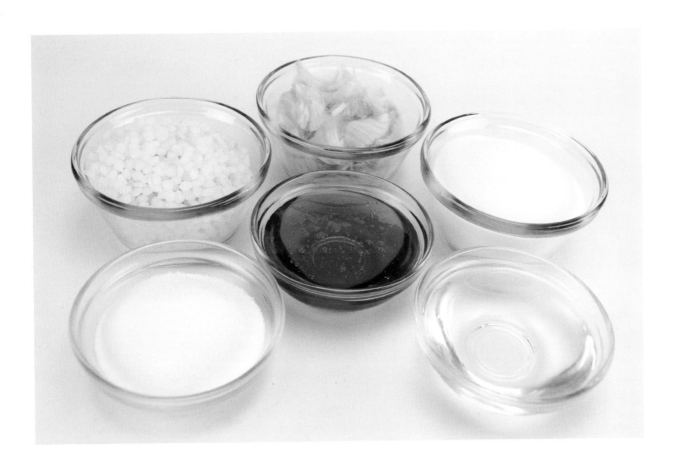

Additives That Are Mostly Just Aesthetic

Flower petals: Rose petals, chamomile, and lavender buds *seem* like beautiful, romantic additions to cold process soap recipes until the soap is unmolded and you realize all the flower petals have turned black. Unfortunately, most all flower petals, *except calendula,* will turn black when they come into contact with lye. Flower petals can be added in hand-milled or rebatched soaps without changing colors—or just know they will change color and create your designs from there. Flower petals, either whole or ground, do give some exfoliation.

Dried leaves, teas, or other plants: Herbs such as rosemary, leaves such as eucalyptus and patchouli, citrus peels, ground rose hips, and teas such as spearmint and peppermint, can all be used to make beautiful soaps. But, like flower petals, they turn brown or black. Most dried leaves, especially rosemary and eucalyptus, need to be ground finely or they can be too scratchy and exfoliating in soap.

A Collection of Basic Soap Recipes

Although formulating your personal favorite soap recipes is one of the most satisfying aspects of making your own soap, most budding soap makers want to jump right in and start. Here is a collection of tried-and-true recipes to try immediately. All the batches of soap in this book (unless specifically noted) were made with one of these recipes. Each is scaled to make 2 pounds (907 g) of soap, but each includes the percentages so you can scale your own recipes.

THE BASIC

I've made hundreds of batches of this recipe over many years. It's a very balanced soap with great lather and moisturizing qualities. The palm and castor oils make it too fast moving to do intricate swirls, but it's just fine for solid colors or basic swirls.

INGREDIENTS

- 7.5 ounces (212.6 g) olive oil (35 percent)
- 6.5 ounces (184 g) palm oil (30 percent)
- 6.5 ounces (184 g) coconut oil (30 percent)
- 1 ounce (28 g) castor oil (5 percent)

- 6.2 ounces (175.8 g) water
- 3.1 ounces (88 g) lye
- 1 ounce (28 g) fragrance oil or essential oil blend

Makes 2 pounds (907 g)

THE BASIC PLUS

To the basic recipe above, this recipe adds sunflower oil, which complements the fatty acids in the palm and olive oils to add creaminess and moisturizing qualities.

INGREDIENTS

- 6.5 ounces (184 g) olive oil (30 percent)
- 6.5 ounces (184 g) coconut oil (30 percent)
- 5.4 ounces (153 g) palm oil (25 percent)
- 2.2 ounces (62 g) sunflower oil (10 percent)

- 1 ounce (31 g) castor oil (5 percent)
- 6.2 ounces (175.8 g) water
- 3 ounces (88 g) lye
- 1 ounce (28 g) fragrance oil or essential oil

Makes 2 pounds (907 g)

A BIT OF LUXURY

This recipe adds cocoa butter, but removes the castor oil, which reduces the bubbles a bit but adds more creaminess to the lather and moisturizing qualities to the soap.

INGREDIENTS

- 6.4 ounces (181.4 g) olive oil (30 percent)
- 5.4 ounces (153 g) coconut oil (25 percent)
- 5.4 ounces (153 g) palm oil (25 percent)
- 3.2 ounces (91 g) sunflower oil (15 percent)

- 1 ounce (28 g) cocoa butter (5 percent)
- 6 ounces (170 g) water
- 3 ounces (85 g) lye
- 1 ounce (28 g) fragrance oil or essential oil blend

Makes 2 pounds (907 g)

THE GROCERY STORE

This is a good basic recipe with ingredients you should be able to get easily at your local grocery store.

INGREDIENTS

- 10.7 ounces (303 g) shortening; make sure it's the new formulation with palm oil (50 percent)
- 5.4 ounces (153 g) olive oil (25 percent)
- 5.4 ounces (153 g) coconut oil (25 percent)
- 3 ounces (85 g) lye
- 6 ounces (170 g) water
- 1 ounce (28 g) fragrance oil or essential oil blend

Makes about 2 pounds (907 g)

THE SLOW MOVER

This recipe was formulated without palm oil or castor oil but, instead, with lard and canola oils to be especially slow to trace. It's a great recipe to use for intricate swirls or creations where you need a lot of time to work with fluid soap batter.

INGREDIENTS

- 6.5 ounces (184 g) olive oil (30 percent)
- 5.4 ounces (153 g) coconut oil (25 percent)
- 3.3 ounces (93.5 g) sunflower oil (15 percent)
- 2.2 ounces (62 g) beef tallow (10 percent)
- 2.2 ounces (62 g) lard (10 percent)
- 2.2 ounces (62 g) canola oil (10 percent)
- 3 ounces (88 g) lye
- 6.2 ounces (175.8 g) water
- 1 ounce (28 g) fragrance oil or essential oil blend

Makes about 2 pounds (907 g)

THE PALM FREE

With the controversies surrounding the production of palm oil, many soap makers have transitioned to recipes that omit it. An easy substitute is either lard or beef tallow, but to stay palm free and not use animal oils, try this recipe that relies on the stearic and palmitic acids in the shea and cocoa butters for hardness. It's also a wonderfully creamy and moisturizing soap.

INGREDIENTS

- 6.4 ounces (181.4 g) olive oil (30 percent)
- 6.4 ounces (181.4 g) coconut oil (30 percent)
- 3.2 ounces (91 g) sunflower oil (15 percent)
- 2 ounces (59.5 g) rice bran oil (10 percent)
- 2 ounces (59.5 g) shea butter (10 percent)
- 1 ounce (28 g) cocoa butter (5 percent)
- 3 ounces (85 g) lye
- 6 ounces (170 g) water
- 1 ounce (28 g) fragrance oil or essential oil blend

Makes about 2 pounds (907 g)

Measurements versus Percentages in Recipes

Most soap recipes are written in one of two ways:

1 In actual measurements:

- 6 ounces (170 g) olive oil
- 6 ounces (170 g) coconut oil
- 5 ounces (141.7 g) palm oil
- 3 ounces (85 g) sunflower oil

2 Or as percentages:

- 30 percent olive oil
- 30 percent coconut oil
- 25 percent palm oil
- 15 percent sunflower oil

Both ways are valuable, but seeing the recipe in percentages allows you to

- Easily scale the recipe to any size mold
- Adjust the balance of the oils to change the qualities of the soap

For example, let's say you have a recipe that makes 2 pounds (907 g) of soap. In it, you might have 5 ounces (142 g) coconut oil. You try the recipe and the lather isn't as good as you'd like, so you want to increase the proportion of coconut oil. With measurements this is difficult, but if you have percentages in addition to the measurements, it's easy.

Converting a Recipe from Measurements to Percentages

We'll start with a simple recipe:

- 6 ounces (170 g) palm oil
- 6 ounces (170 g) coconut oil
- 7 ounces (198.5 g) olive oil
- 1 ounce (28 g) castor oil

This will make a 2-pound (907 g) batch of soap. But what are the ratios of each oil? Is this a well-balanced recipe? And what if you want to make 7 pounds (3.2 kg) of soap?

Here's what you do:

1 Total the number of ounces (grams) of oils. In this case, the ounces total 20 (6 + 6 + 7 + 1); the gram total is 566.5.

2 Divide each individual ounce weight by the total ounces, 20 (or total grams: 566.5), to get the percentage of that oil in the recipe.

So:

- 6 ounces (170 g) palm oil ÷ 20 = 30 (0.30) percent or 170 ÷ 566.5 = 30 (0.30) percent
- 6 ounces (170 g) coconut oil ÷ 20 = 30 (0.30) percent or 170 ÷ 566.5 = 30 (0.30) percent
- 7 ounces (198.5 g) olive oil ÷ 20 = 35 (0.35) percent or 198.5 ÷ 566.5 = 35 (0.35) percent
- 1 ounce (28 g) castor oil ÷ 20 = 5 (0.05) percent or 28 ÷ 566.5 = 5 (0.05) percent

So, your recipe is

- 30 percent palm oil
- 30 percent coconut oil
- 35 percent olive oil
- 5 percent castor oil

A well-balanced recipe.

To convert this recipe into a larger-scale recipe, use the percentages and multiply by the total amount of oils in the new batch. A 10-pound (4.5 kg) batch would have about 112 ounces (3.17 kg) of oils in it. To scale your recipe up to that:

- 30 percent (0.30) palm oil × 112 ounces (or 3,175 g) = 33.6 ounces (or 952.5 g)
- 30 percent (0.30) coconut oil × 112 (or 3,175 g) = 33.6 ounces (or 952.5 g)
- 35 percent (0.35) olive oil × 112 ounces (or 3,175 g) = 39.2 ounces (or 1 kg)
- 5 percent (0.05) castor oil × 112 (or 3,175 g) = 5.6 ounces (or 158.8 g)

Online lye calculators can calculate most of this for you, but they cannot make the fine adjustments you want to make in your recipes. That is the most valuable benefit of percentages, allowing you to adjust the ratio of each oil in your soap to produce the exact qualities—hard, creamy, bubbly, or moisturizing—you want in your soap.

Mixing It Up: Adding Color and More to Your Cold Process Soap

The place to start adding color to your soap is right in the soap batter—right after you've reached light trace. However, you don't just have to make the color uniform throughout. It's easy to do swirls right in the pot or whatever vessel you are mixing your soap in.

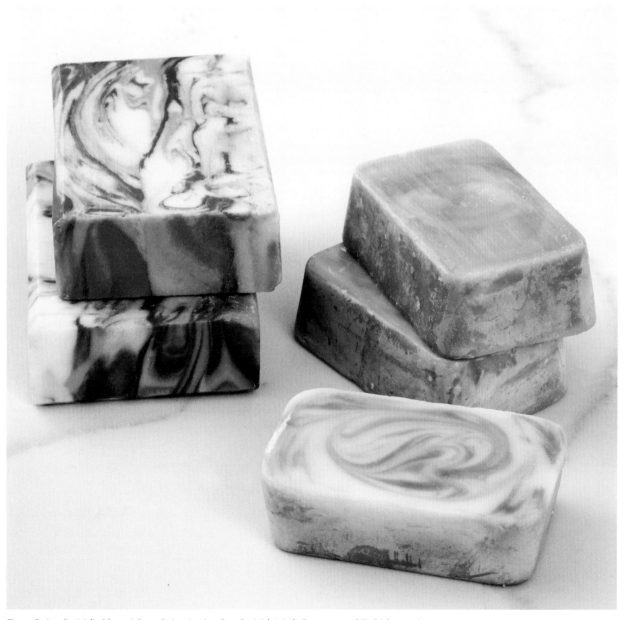

Four-Color Swirl (left) and One Color in-the-Pot Swirl (right). See pages 90–91 for recipes.

In-the-Pot Soap Swirls

ONE COLOR IN-THE-POT SWIRL

Start with the basic soap recipe (page 86) and follow standard soap-making procedures for this recipe.

1 In the large measuring cup, whisk the colorant with 1 tablespoon (15 ml) melted soap oils (A).

2 When the soap is fully mixed and at light to medium trace, pour about one-third of the soap batter into the measuring cup with the colorant (B). Whisk to incorporate fully.

3 Pour the colored soap back into the pot in a circular and/or zigzag motion, varying the height of the pour to make some of the color go deep to the bottom of the pot, and some of it stay shallow near the top (C).

INGREDIENTS

- 1 teaspoon mica or oxide, or natural soap colorant

EQUIPMENT

- Large measuring cup
- Your main soap pot
- Chopstick or small spatula

Makes 2 pounds (907 g)

4 Using a chopstick or small spatula, swirl the soap in a circle once or twice (D). (For a more mixed swirl effect, swirl across the pot as well.)

5 Pour the soap batter into a loaf or individual molds (E).

6 If desired, swirl the soaps once more in the molds (F).

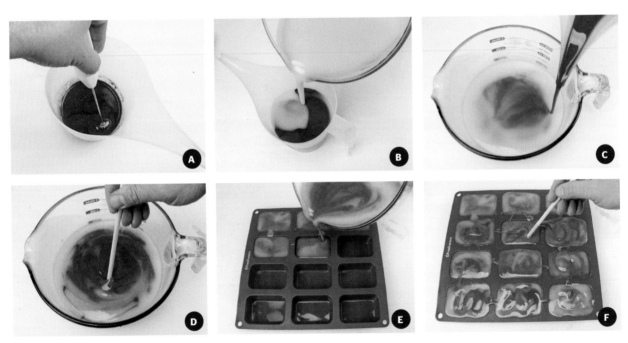

See page 89 for the finished soap.

FOUR-COLOR SWIRL

This recipe works the same as the One Color in-the-Pot Swirl (page 90) but, instead, separates the soap into three additional colors.

Start with the Basic Plus (page 86) soap recipe and follow standard soap-making procedures for this recipe.

1 Follow the directions for the One Color in-the-Pot Swirl (page 90) but prepare four colors in separate measuring cups (A).

2 Place the titanium dioxide in a small ramekin and mix with 1 to 2 tablespoons (15 to 30 ml) of melted oils.

3 When the soap is fully mixed and is at light to medium trace, pour about 4 to 6 ounces (113 to 170 g) of soap batter into each of the measuring cups with the colorants. Whisk to incorporate the colorants fully. You will have 4 containers with about 4 to 6 ounces (113 to 170 g) colored soap, and the remaining uncolored soap still in the pot.

4 Add the titanium dioxide mixture to the remaining soap in the pot and mix to combine (B).

5 Pour the four colors back into the main soap pot in four places: top, bottom, left, and right (C).

6 Using a chopstick or small spatula, swirl the soap in a circle once or twice (D). (For a more mixed swirl effect, swirl across the pot as well.)

7 Pour the soap batter into a loaf or individual molds (E).

8 If desired, swirl the top 0.5 inch (1 cm) of soap in the mold with a chopstick (F).

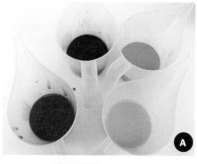
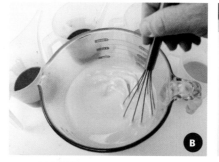
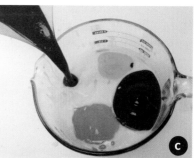
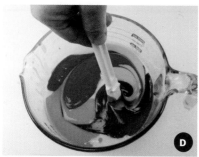
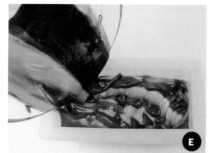
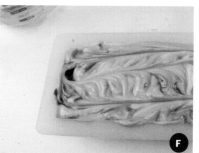

See page 89 for the finished soap.

In-the-Mold Swirls

Even more complex designs can be created by separating portions of soap batter, coloring them, and layering and swirling the soap batter in the mold. There are many assorted designs, techniques, and styles—all make great soap. The only limit is your imagination and the time it takes before the soap batter starts to thicken.

SPOON PLOP PATTERN SOAP

INGREDIENTS
- ½ teaspoon each of five different micas

EQUIPMENT
- 5 large measuring cups or bowls
- Large spoon (tablespoon or larger)
- Chopstick

Makes 2 pounds (907 g)

This is a great starter project to incorporate layered colors in the soap because it takes advantage of recipes that may go to trace quickly. (It's also a good technique for all soap makers to have in their back pocket, just in case that batch you wanted to do a complex swirl in suddenly thickens!)

Start with the basic soap recipe (page 86) and follow standard soap-making procedures for this recipe.

1 In each measuring cup, whisk one of the micas with 1 tablespoon (15 ml) melted soap oils (A).

2 When the soap is fully mixed and is at light trace, pour equal amounts into each measuring cup and whisk to incorporate the colorants fully (B). Keep mixing the soap batter until it is at medium trace. This is necessary for the dollops of soap to hold up.

3 Using the large spoon, scoop a dollop of soap from one measuring cup into the mold (C).

4 Alternate with each color, filling the mold from end to end (D). Tap the mold on the counter after every inch (2.5 cm) or so of soap is placed into the mold. Leave just a bit of soap in each container.

5 Drizzle the remaining soap onto the top of the full soap mold (E).

6 Insert a chopstick about 0.5 inch (1 cm) into the soap and draw a zigzag line back and forth along the width of the mold to swirl the top of the soap (F).

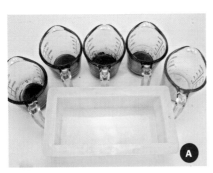
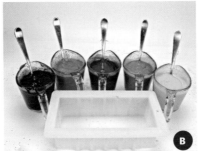
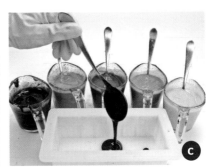
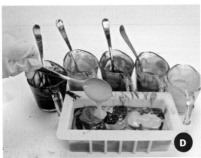
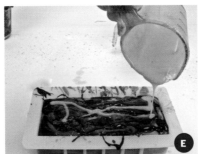
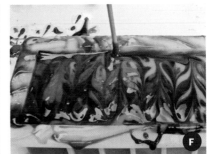

SIX-COLOR SQUIRTY LAYERED SOAP

This soap project layers the soap into the mold like the Spoon Plop Pattern Soap (page 90), but uses squirt bottles, which leave small, random lines of soap color.

Start with a slow-moving soap recipe, such as the Slow Mover (page 87) and follow basic soap-making procedures for this recipe.

INGREDIENTS
- ½ teaspoon each of six micas or titanium dioxide

EQUIPMENT
- 6 large squirt bottles
- Chopstick

Makes 1 (4-pound or 1.8 kg) loaf

1. In each squirt bottle, mix one mica with 1 tablespoon (15 ml) melted soap oils (A). Replace the tops. Hold your finger over the tip of a bottle and shake vigorously. Repeat until all bottles have been shaken.

2. When the soap is just fully emulsified (very light trace), pour equal amounts into the 6 bottles and shake again to incorporate the colorant fully.

3. Once mixed, squirt a line of 1 color of soap down the middle of the mold's length (B). If the line holds its shape, or sags just a little, the soap is thick enough. If the soap spreads, shake the bottles again until the soap thickens a bit.

4. Continue squirting lines of soap in the same direction along the bottom of the mold (C). After each color of soap is put into the mold, tap the mold on the counter to help the soap settle.

5. Continue squirting the soap lines until the mold is full.

6. Insert a chopstick about 0.5 inch (1 cm) into the soap and draw a zigzag line back and forth along the width of the mold to swirl the top of the soap (D).

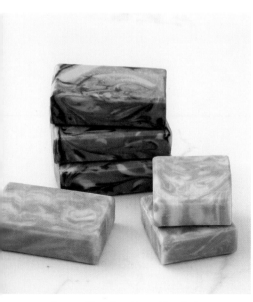

Spoon Plop (back) and Six-Color Squirty layered (front) soaps.

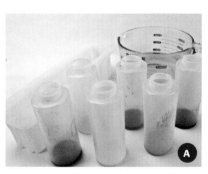
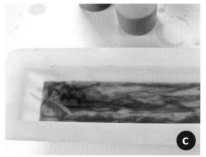
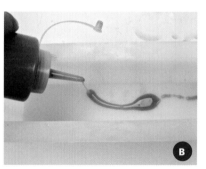
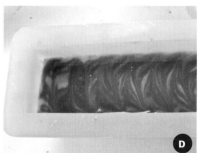

HANGER SWIRLS

Many different utensils can be used to swirl soap—chopsticks, rubber spatulas, spoons—but a plain piece of wire, bent to the size of your mold, makes wonderful swirls in loaf molds.

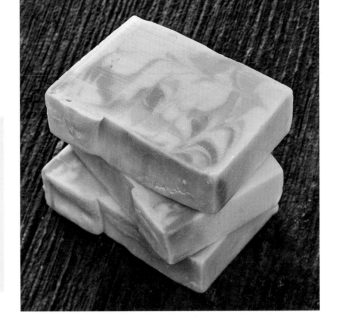

INGREDIENTS

- ½ teaspoon green mica
- ½ teaspoon yellow mica
- 1 teaspoon titanium dioxide

Makes 2 pounds (907 g)

EQUIPMENT

- 2 large measuring cups
- Small ramekin
- Hanger swirl tool

Start with a soap recipe such as A Bit of Luxury (page 86).

1 In each measuring cup, whisk 1 mica with 1 tablespoon (15 ml) melted soap oils.

2 Mix the titanium dioxide with 2 tablespoons (30 ml) melted oils in the ramekin.

3 When the soap is fully mixed and is at light trace, divide half the soap between the 2 measuring cups and whisk to incorporate the mica fully.

4 Add the titanium dioxide to the rest of the batch in the pot.

5 Pour the two different soap colors and the remaining white soap in layers into the mold (A), alternating colors until the mold is full (B).

6 Move the hanger swirl tool through the soap (C) using one of the hanger swirl patterns shown (see page 95). This one uses pattern 1—an up-and-down movement.

7 Swirl the top 0.5 inch (1 cm) of the soap with a chopstick (if desired).

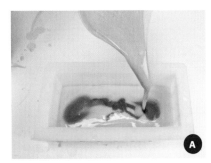
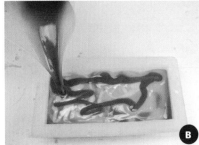
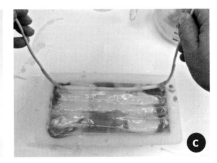

Try one of these hanger swirl patterns or create your own.

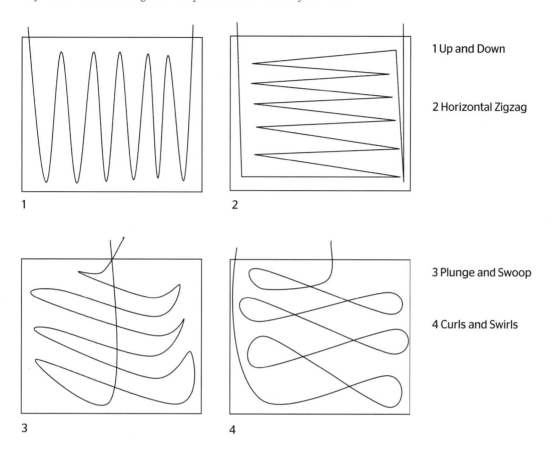

1 Up and Down

2 Horizontal Zigzag

3 Plunge and Swoop

4 Curls and Swirls

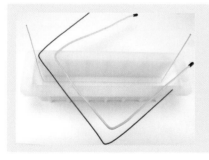

How to Make a Hanger Swirl Tool

To make a reusable hanger swirl tool, use a length of 10G coated copper wire. And, just like the size difference between a chopstick and a spatula gives different swirl effects, using different thicknesses of wire does the same. Try covering your wire with a length of aquarium tubing or even thicker rubber hose to make a more dramatic hanger swirl.

Slab Mold Swirls

Slab molds make large, flat slabs of soap, so the orientation is different than a loaf mold. Because you are looking at the soap at only one bar's worth of thickness, you can see the swirls you are creating.

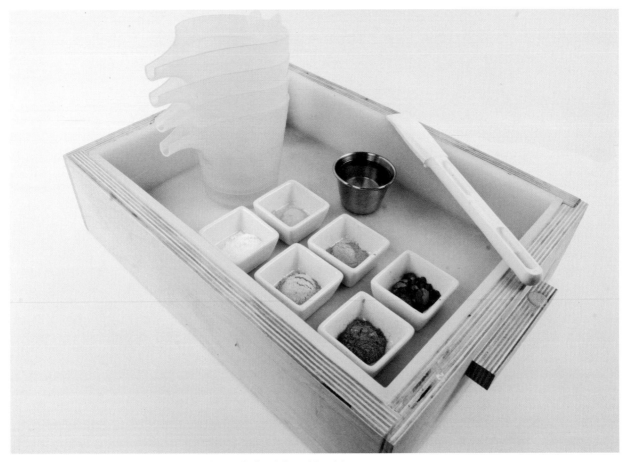

Micas, measuring cups, fragrance oil, and spatula for slab mold swirl.

BASIC FREE-FORM SLAB MOLD SWIRL

Start with a soap recipe such as the Slow Mover (page 87; scaled to 4.5 pounds [2 kg])—you'll need lots of time to manipulate the soap!—and follow standard soap-making procedures for this recipe.

1 In each measuring cup, whisk 1 teaspoon of one of the micas with 1 tablespoon (15 ml) melted soap oils.

2 Add the fragrance oil to the melted oils and then mix the lye and oils just until fully emulsified (a very light trace).

INGREDIENTS
- ½ to 1 teaspoon each of 6 different micas

EQUIPMENT
- 6 large measuring cups
- Slab mold
- Small rubber spatula or chopstick

Makes 4.5 pounds (2 kg)

3 Divide the soap evenly among the measuring cups. Stir until the colors are well blended with the soap (A).

4 Starting with whichever color you want, pour the soap in a zigzag line across the bottom of the mold (B). Select the next color and pour some on top of the first layer (C).

5 Continue rotating through the colors, adding a layer at a time. You can zigzag the soap or pour it in straight lines or in circles (D). Each gives a different effect when you cut the final bars. Tap the mold gently on the counter after each inch (2.5 cm) of soap is put into the mold.

6 Use a chopstick or small spatula to swirl it—inserting it all the way to the bottom of one corner of the mold and dragging it through the soap in a back-and-forth zigzag motion going from one end of the mold to the other (E).

7 Repeat the zigzag motion in the other direction, crossing your original lines (F). How much or little you swirl, and whether in a pattern or free-form is entirely up to you.

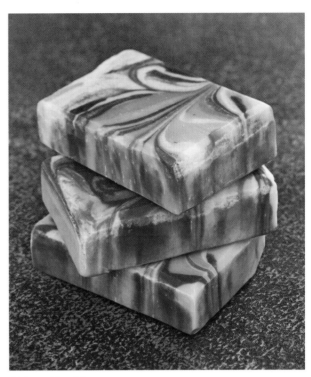

Slab mold swirl.

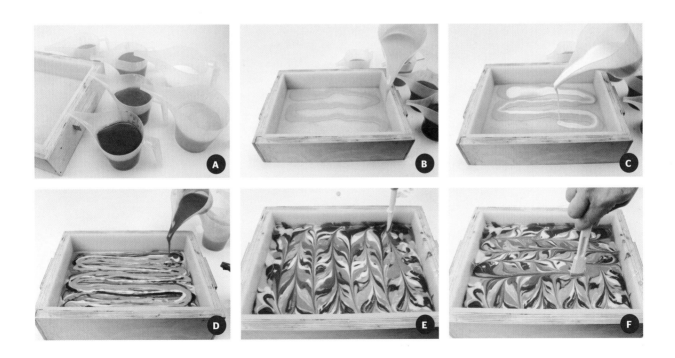

FUNNEL POUR IN SLAB MOLD

Funnel pour swirls use a simple kitchen funnel to direct the soap in one multiringed layer like the rings on a growing tree.

Start with a soap recipe such as the Slow Mover (page 87; scaled to 3 pounds [1.3 kg]) and follow standard soap-making procedures for this recipe.

1 In each measuring cup, whisk 1 mica with 1 tablespoon (15 ml) melted soap oils.

2 Add the fragrance oil to the melted oils and then mix the lye and oils just until fully emulsified (a very light trace).

3 Divide the soap evenly among the measuring cups. Stir the colored soap so it's well blended.

4 Hold the funnel about 2 inches (5 cm) above one corner of the slab mold. Pour a few ounces (g) of one color into the funnel and let it run down into the mold (A).

5 Repeat with the remaining colors, pouring a few ounces (about 85 g) each time (B).

6 Repeat until all the soap is poured into the mold (C and D).

7 Leave the ringed swirl effect or use a chopstick or small spatula to swirl, inserting it to the bottom of the mold's corner you poured from, and dragging it through the soap in a back-and-forth zigzag motion (E).

8 For even more swirl effect, drag through the swirls in a free-form motion (F).

INGREDIENTS
- ½ to 1 teaspoon each of 5 different micas

EQUIPMENT
- 5 large measuring cups
- Funnel
- Slab mold
- Small rubber spatula or chopstick

Makes 3 pounds (1.3 kg)

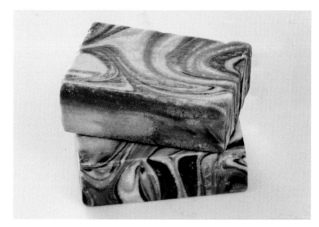

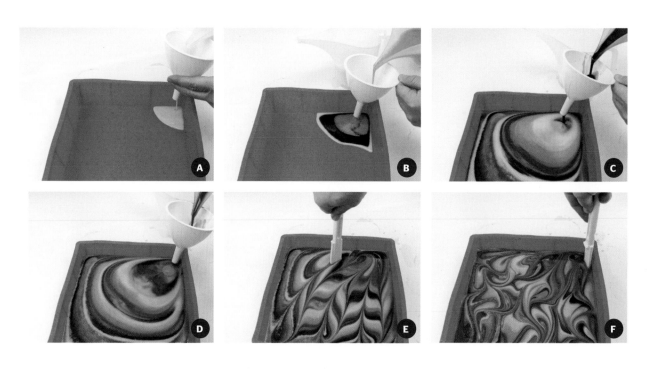

MANTRA SWIRL

This popular swirl uses a simple swirled back-and-forth motion, but it divides the soap with cardboard dividers to separate the colors. It also (to show the full effect) requires that you cut the soap horizontally rather than vertically.

Start with a recipe such as the Slow Mover (page 87; scaled to 4 pounds [1.8kg]) and follow standard soap-making procedures for this recipe.

You will need an extra set of hands—*a soap helper*—for this recipe to help hold the dividers in place while you pour the soap. Be sure your helper is also wearing gloves and goggles.

INGREDIENTS
- 1 teaspoon green mica
- 1 teaspoon blue mica
- 1 teaspoon titanium dioxide

EQUIPMENT
- 3 medium-size measuring cups
- 3 cardboard dividers snugly cut to the length of your soap mold and 2 inches (5 cm) taller than the depth of your mold
- Chopstick

Makes 4 pounds (1.8 kg)

1. In each measuring cup, whisk one colorant with 2 tablespoons (30 ml) melted soap oils.

2. Set the cardboard dividers into the mold (A).

3. Add the fragrance oil to the melted oils and then mix the lye and oils just until fully emulsified (a very light trace). Divide the soap evenly among the three containers. Whisk the colorant into the soap well.

4. Using a soap helper, pour three portions of soap slowly and simultaneously into the three sections of the mold. An extra hand is good to hold the dividers (B).

5. When all the soap is in the mold, slowly pull the dividers straight up and out of the mold (C).

6. Using a chopstick, make a left and right figure-eight motion, going straight down to the bottom of the mold (D).

7. Make one move around the perimeter of the mold.

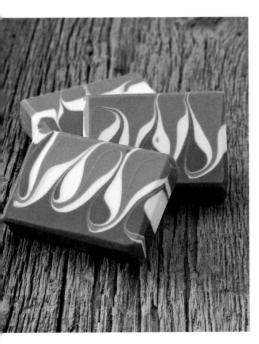

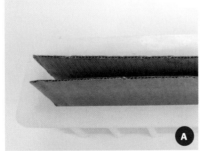

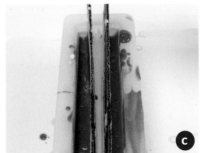

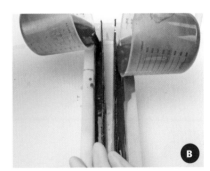

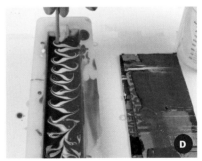

DOT SWIRL SOAP

The Dot Swirl uses squeeze bottles like the Six-Color Squirty Layered Soap (page 93) but, instead of back-and-forth lines of soap, creates round soap dots randomly layered on top of each other. The effect is a wonderful collection of random curved designs that are different in each bar and change as the soap is used.

Start with a slow-moving recipe such as the Slow Mover (page 87; scaled to 4.5 pounds [2 kg]) and follow standard soap-making procedures for this recipe.

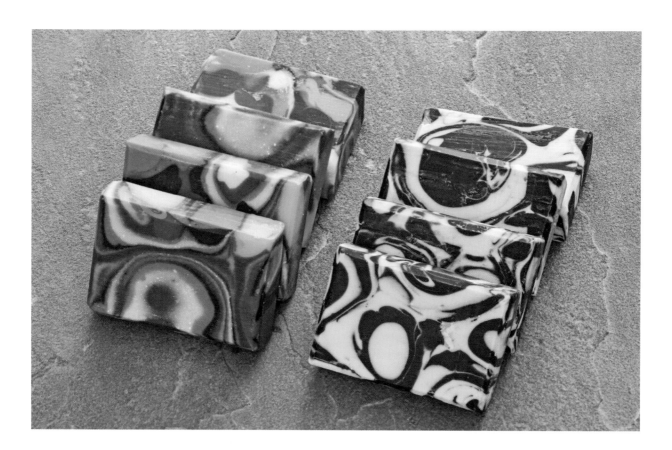

INGREDIENTS

- 2 teaspoons activated charcoal
- 2 teaspoons titanium dioxide

EQUIPMENT

- 2 small measuring cups or ramekins
- Large container to hold half the soap
- Slab mold
- 2 large squirt bottles

Makes 4.5 pounds (2 kg)

1 In each measuring cup, whisk 1 colorant with 2 tablespoons (30 ml) melted soap oils.

2 After mixing in the fragrance as noted in the recipe, separate half the soap into another container and add the black colorant to it. Stir to blend well.

3 Add the titanium dioxide to the remaining soap. Stir to blend well.

4 Pour each color into a squirt bottle (A).

5 With one color, make dots of soap that cover the bottom of the mold (B).

6 With the second color, make dots of soap on top of the existing dots, and in between the dots, as well (C).

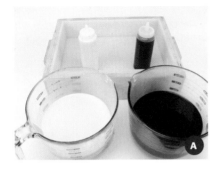

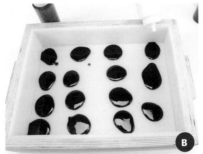

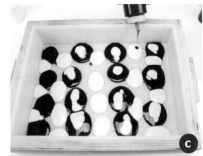

7 Continue switching colors, placing dots of soap on top of and in between the existing dots (D). Tap the mold on the counter frequently to settle the soap in the mold.

8 Continue making dots of soap until all the soap is in the mold (E).

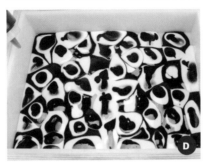

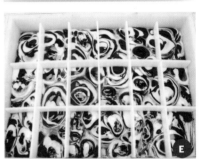

Dot Swirl Variation: Faux Funnel Pour

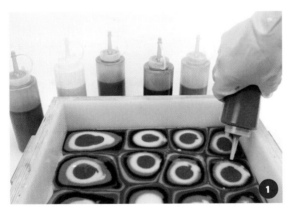

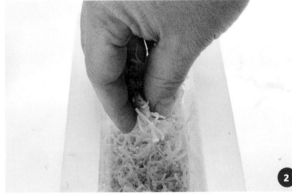

1 Prepare multiple colors of soap in squirt bottles and make dots of soap in the mold. However, instead of putting the dots both on top of and in between each other, put them only on top of each other, like a funnel pour (see page 98).

2 Keep making funnel pour dots, or, after the bottom of the mold is covered with dots, create layers of random dots, placing dots of soap in between the funnel-ring circles.

SPRING FLOWERS SHREDS SOAP

For this recipe, we'll use two kinds of shreds to create a flower-like design in the loaf of soap.

Start with the Basic soap recipe (page 86; scaled to 4 pounds [1.8 kg]) and follow standard soap-making procedures for this recipe.

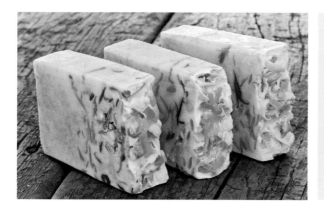

INGREDIENTS
- 10 ounces (283.5 g) light green fine soap shreds
- 10 ounces (283.5 g) multicolored coarse soap shreds

EQUIPMENT
- Tall soap mold

Makes about 4 pounds (1.8 kg)

1 Place 0.5 to 0.75 inch (1 to 2 cm) fine light green soap shreds into the bottom of the soap mold (A).

2 Make the scaled batch of the basic soap, adding any desired fragrance or color, and bringing it to light trace.

3 Pour enough fresh soap into the mold to barely cover the light green shreds (B).

4 Add another 0.5 to 0.75 inch (1 to 2 cm) of light green soap shreds, concentrating them in the middle of the mold like the stem of a flower (C).

5 Pour enough fresh soap into the mold to cover the light green shreds. Repeat steps 4 and 5 until you have filled about two-thirds of the mold.

6 Place 0.25 inch (0.6 cm) of multicolored soap shreds into the middle of the mold, just above the light green shreds (D).

7 Add another 0.25 inch (0.6 cm) of multicolored soap shreds in a slightly wider pattern, and overpour with the fresh soap.

8 Continue placing more multicolored shreds, arranging them in a wider and wider pattern, and overpouring with fresh soap until they span the whole width of the mold and you have filled the mold with the remaining overpour (E).

9 Sprinkle a bit more colored soap shreds on the top and gently push them into the top of the soap (F).

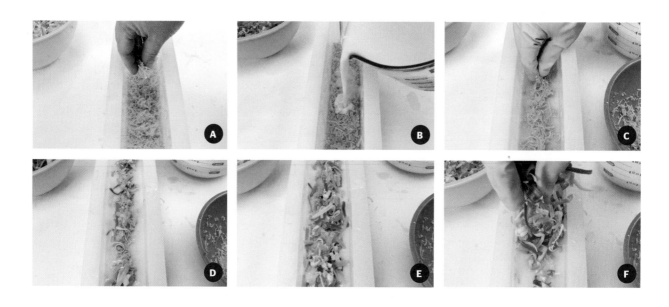

LAYERED HEART EMBED SOAP

This recipe uses a layered technique with a mica line and an embedded premade soap shape.
Start with the Basic soap recipe (page 86) and follow standard soap-making procedures for this recipe.

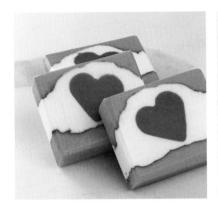

INGREDIENTS
- Premade heart embed cut to the horizontal length of your mold (see step 1)
- ½ teaspoon pink mica
- ½ teaspoon titanium dioxide
- 1 to 2 teaspoons burgundy mica

EQUIPMENT
- Tea ball or other tea steeper
- 1 (2 pounds or 907 g) soap mold
- 2 large measuring cups
- Ramekin

Makes 2 pounds (907 kg)

1 Make the heart-shaped embed using a plastic or silicone tube mold. You can make this out of melt-and-pour soap, a small cold process batch, or from a bit of leftover soap. Subtract its weight from the total weight of the soap loaf you are going to make and scale the recipe properly. (Or just know you'll have soap left over and have ready a couple of small individual molds.)

2 In a measuring cup, mix the pink mica with 2 tablespoons (30 ml) melted soap oils.

3 Mix the titanium dioxide with 2 tablespoons (30 ml) of melted soap oil.

4 Scoop 1 teaspoon of burgundy mica into the tea strainer.

5 Make the scaled batch of fresh soap, adding the fragrance and bringing it to light trace.

6 Mix half the soap with the pink mica and the other half with the titanium dioxide.

7 Pour half the pink soap into the mold.

8 Lightly dust the top of the pink soap with the burgundy mica by gently tapping on the tea ball (A).

9 Close your eyes, move about 8 inches (20 cm) away from the soap and gently blow on the mica to distribute it evenly on the soap.

10 Pour about 0.5 inch (1 cm) of white soap over a spatula on top of the mica-dusted soap layer (B).

11 Place the heart embed into the white soap and push it down just enough to ensure no air bubbles are below it. **Note:** You'll notice I put the heart in upside down. I did this to ensure the pointy part of the heart wouldn't sink into the layer, but, rather, the larger surface area of the top of the heart is better supported.

12 Pour the remaining white soap over the embed.

13 Dust the white soap layer with the burgundy mica as in steps 8 and 9.

14 Pour the remaining pink soap over a spatula into the mold.

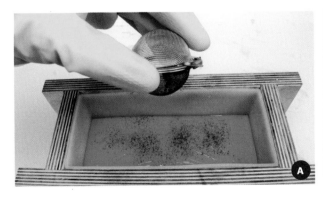

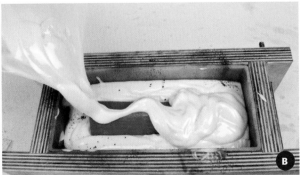

Using Milk in Soap Recipes

In addition to adding interest and creativity to your soap making, using a liquid other than water to make your soap is an effective way to add moisturizing or lathering qualities to the soap. Milk, in particular goat's milk, is one of the most popular alternate liquids used in soap.

Goat's milk producers and soap makers generally give two primary reasons why it makes great soap:

1   The vitamins, minerals, caseins, and proteins in the milk (some of which survive the saponification process) are known to be moisturizing, soothing, and exfoliating for your skin.

2   The added fat in the milk makes the soap milder and more moisturizing.

In addition to goat's milk, other types of milk—animal and vegetable—can be used in soap. Each will impart its own unique constituents to the recipe. Unless you decrease the superfat of your recipe to compensate for the milk, the milk will add a bit of extra fat to the soap. The naturally occurring sugars in the milk also help boost the soap's lather. Below are the methods to add milk to your soap:.

1   Use frozen milk (fresh or condensed)

2   Use powdered milk

3   Use fresh milk, added to the oils

While the results are quite similar, each requires a slightly different technique to add the milk.

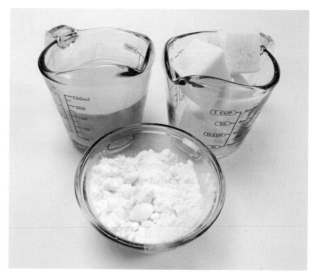

Clockwise from upper left: canned goat's milk, frozen heavy cream, and powered goat's milk.

How Much Milk?

Milk is a wonderful additive to include in soap recipes, but with the different methods of adding it, how much is the right amount? A good rule of thumb is up to 100 percent of the water in the recipe.

* If using fresh milk, just substitute the milk for the water.
* If using powdered milk, use as much powder as would be needed to make enough regular strength milk to substitute for the water.
* If using condensed milk, use half milk and half water to bring it to regular strength.

Less than 100 percent can be used as well, especially with powdered or condensed milks that you add to the oils or at trace.

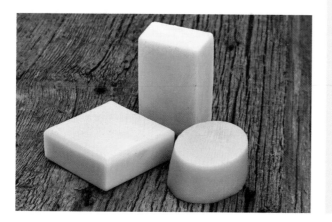

GOAT'S MILK SOAP USING FROZEN MILK

This recipe uses frozen, regular strength goat's milk. (Any other type of regular or condensed milk can be substituted.)

Start with the Basic soap recipe (page 86) and follow basic soap-making procedures for this recipe.

1 Freeze the milk in ice cube trays (A).

2 Weigh the appropriate amount of milk cubes (up to 100 percent) to replace the water in your soap recipe and place it in the lye pitcher.

3 Slowly . . . very slowly . . . add a bit of the lye to the frozen milk (B). The lye will begin to react with the water in the milk and heat up, melting the milk cubes.

4 Gently stir the lye and frozen milk (C). The objective is to keep the lye-milk cool.

5 After 1 to 2 minutes, add a bit more lye and repeat until it is all added, patiently waiting and stirring as the milk continues to melt and combine with the lye, but never gets hot enough to scorch (D).

6 Mix the lye-milk solution with the oils and blend to trace (E).

INGREDIENTS

- Lye solution made with frozen milk instead of water (see Note)

EQUIPMENT

- Ice cube trays
- Pitcher, for the lye solution
- Loaf mold or individual soap molds

Makes 2 pounds (907 g)

7 Pour the soap batter into the mold(s). To keep it as white as possible, you don't want this soap to get too hot and go through a gel stage. If using a loaf mold, keep it in a cool place and do not cover it with a towel. If using individual molds, just cover with a light towel.

Note: Remember that a lye solution will reach 200°F (93°C) or higher when it is mixed. If fresh milk is combined with the lye at room temperature, and gets that hot, the sugars in the milk will scorch, turn a bright orange or brown color, and often smell bad. The final soap will have a beige color, but the smell will go away.

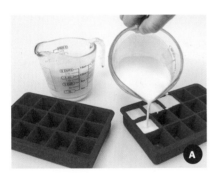
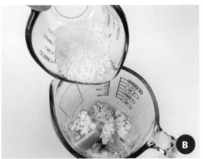
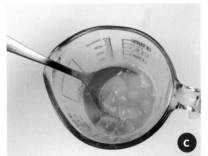
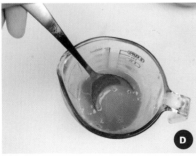
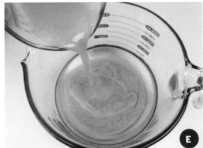

COCONUT MILK SOAP WITH POWDERED MILK

Like coconut oil, coconut milk gives a boost to the lather in the soap. Canned, liquid coconut milk can be used, or powdered milk is a very easy option to add the benefits of milk without the need to make the special frozen-milk lye solution.

Start with the Basic soap recipe (page 86) and follow basic soap-making procedures for this recipe.

1 Mix the coconut milk powder with enough water to make a light slurry (A). Subtract this amount of water from the amount you use to make your lye solution.

2 Add the coconut milk slurry directly to the oils (B), or add it at trace.

3 Mix the lye solution with the oils and blend to trace.

4 Add fragrance and any color as desired.

5 Pour the soap batter into the mold(s) (C).

INGREDIENTS
- Coconut milk powder equal to the amount needed to make enough regular strength milk to substitute for the water in the batch

EQUIPMENT
- Loaf mold or individual soap molds

Makes 2 pounds (907 kg)

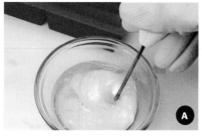 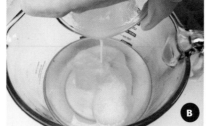 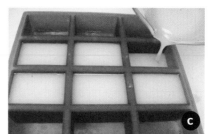

BUTTERMILK SOAP USING MILK IN OILS

This method uses the milk-in-oils technique, which can be done with fresh or condensed milk. Making the lye solution is more difficult, but as the milk is added directly to the oils, very little scorching or color shift occurs. Using condensed milk, you can add enough to make 100 percent of the lye solution. Using fresh milk, you are only going to substitute 50 percent of the water in the lye solution for milk.

Start with the Basic soap recipe (page 86) and follow basic soap-making procedures for this recipe.

1 Using extra caution, make the 1 : 1 lye solution and stir. *If the lye does not fully dissolve, add a bit more water, 1 tablespoon (15 ml) at a time, until it is fully dissolved.

2 Add the buttermilk to the melted soap oils and blend (A).

3 Mix the lye solution with the oils and blend to trace.

4 Add fragrance or color as desired.

5 Pour the soap batter into the mold(s) (B).

INGREDIENTS
- 1 : 1 lye and water solution (see step 1)
- 1 part buttermilk equal to the amount of water (see Note, opposite)

EQUIPMENT
- Loaf mold or individual soap molds

Makes 2 pounds (907 g)

6 As with the goat's milk soap (see page 105), to keep it as white as possible, you don't want this soap to get too hot and go through a gel stage. If using a loaf mold, keep it in a cool place and do not cover it with a towel. If using individual molds, just cover with a light towel.

Note: In a recipe that uses 3 ounces (88 g) of lye, you would make the lye solution with 3 ounces (88 g) water and add 3 ounces (88 g) milk to the oils.

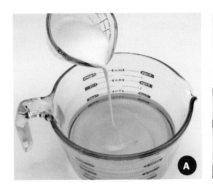
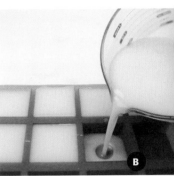

Making Soap with Liquids Other Than Milk

Although milk may be one of the most popular substitutes for water in soap recipes, most any liquid you can drink can be substituted, including juices, teas, beer, and wine.

Using Alcohol-Containing Liquids in Soap Recipes

Alcohol reacts poorly with the saponification process, so the alcohol must be cooked out of liquids that contain it. In addition, carbonation can cause the lye-liquid reaction to be volatile, like opening a shaken can of soda.

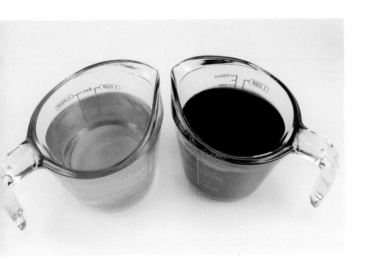

To make soap with beer or wine:

1 Measure at least *twice* the amount of liquid you'll need for your recipe. (The beer or wine will cook down as it simmers. If you end up cooking off too much water, you can add some water when making your lye solution.)

2 Simmer it over low heat for 15 to 20 minutes until all the carbonation (in the case of beer) is removed.

3 Refrigerate it to cool, or freeze it into cubes.

4 **Do not** mix lye with the hot liquid! You'll create a hot, bubbly beer and lye volcano!

Bubbly Beer Soaps

AMBER BEER SOAP AND BLACK ALE SOAP

Start with a soap recipe such as the Palm Free (page 87) and follow standard soap-making procedures for this recipe.

1 Boil the beer at a low simmer for 20 to 30 minutes to remove the alcohol and carbonation. Freeze the beer into cubes.

2 Slowly make the lye solution with the beer cubes and set aside (A).

3 In the measuring cup, whisk the mica with 2 tablespoons (30 ml) soap oils.

4 Add the lye solution to the oils and blend to trace (B).

5 Add the fragrance oil.

6 Mix one third of the soap batch with the mica.

7 Pour the colored soap back into the soap pot (C) and pour it into the molds (D).

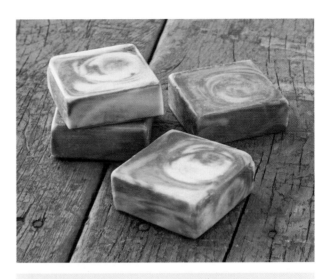

INGREDIENTS

- Beer (double the amount needed to replace the water; It will reduce as it boils)
- ½ teaspoon mica, for swirl

EQUIPMENT

- Ice cube trays
- Measuring cup

Makes 2 pounds (907 g)

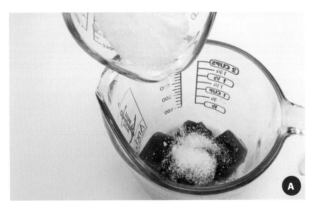

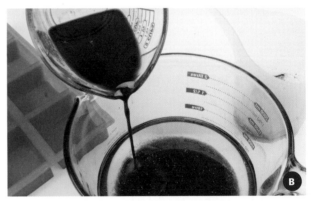

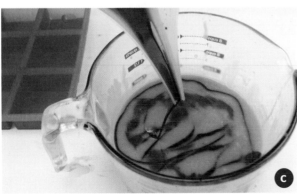

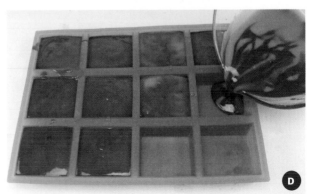

Wonderful Wine Soaps

These soaps have no added color to them—the only color is that imparted by the wine.

Start with a soap recipe such as the Grocery Store (page 87) and follow standard soap-making procedures for this recipe.

1 Boil the wine at a low simmer for 20 to 30 minutes to remove the alcohol.

2 Freeze the wine into cubes.

3 Weigh out frozen wine cubes equal to the amount of water in your recipe. As with other frozen liquids, slowly make the lye solution with the frozen wine and set aside.

4 Add the lye solution to the oils and blend to trace.

5 Add the fragrance oil.

6 Pour the mixed soap into the molds.

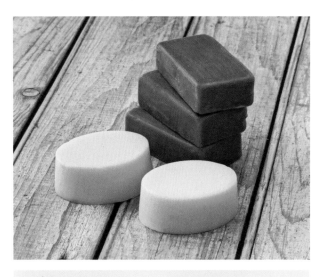

INGREDIENTS
- Wine (start out with double the amount needed to replace the water; it will reduce as it boils)

EQUIPMENT
- Ice cube trays
- Soap molds

Makes 2 pounds (907 g)

Making Soap with Juices

Pretty much anything that can be reduced to a liquid juice can be used in soap. Fruit juices, such as orange, berry, and mango, and vegetable juices, such as carrot, cucumber, beet, and wheatgrass, can all be used in soap. Most fruit juices will add sugar, which will boost lather. Most other plants and vegetables will add only water and, sometimes, color, though aloe vera juice can be used in soap and is reputed to bring some of its moisturizing qualities to the soap.

To make soap with juice:

- **Option 1:** Refrigerate the juice to cool before using it to make a lye solution, or freeze it into cubes.

- **Option 2:** Make a more concentrated purée out of the fruit or vegetable and use it like a double-strength milk, reducing the amount of water in the lye solution by up to half, and adding the purée to the oils before the lye solution is added.

Soaps Made with Tea

Tea can be used as an additive in cold process soap, both the liquid as a water substitute and the leaves as a botanical and light exfoliant.

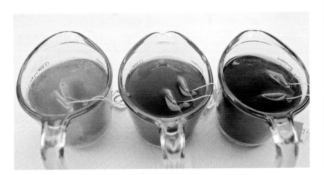

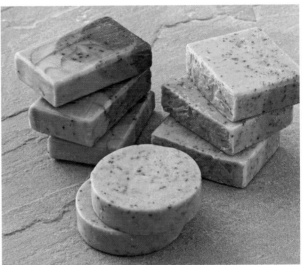

ROSE CLAY AND RED ROOIBOS TEA SOAP

This simple soap (use a recipe of your choosing) uses red rooibos tea as a substitute for the water and adds rose clay and the tea leaves for color and exfoliation into cubes. (The finished soap is shown above, in the foreground.)

1 Make the lye solution: Add the lye to the frozen tea cubes as you would with any other frozen liquid (see page 105).

2 Disperse the rose clay and the tea leaves in 2 tablespoons (30 ml) melted soap oils.

3 Mix the lye with the oils and bring to light trace.

4 Blend in the fragrance oil, clay, and tea leaves.

5 Pour the soap into the molds.

INGREDIENTS

- Double-strength brewed red rooibos tea (in an amount equal to replace the water), frozen into cubes
- 1 tablespoon (14 g) brewed tea leaves per 1 lb (454 g) of soap
- 1 teaspoon rose clay per 1 lb (454 g) of soap

EQUIPMENT

- Soap molds

Yield: Varies

CHAI TEA SOAP WITH MANTRA SWIRL

This recipe uses the tea leaves and micas in a Mantra Swirl (page 99).

Start with a slow-moving recipe such as the Palm Free (page 87) and follow standard soap-making procedures for this recipe. (The finished soap is shown above, top left.)

INGREDIENTS

- Double-strength brewed chai tea (in an equal amount to replace the water), frozen into cubes
- 2 tablespoons (28 g) brewed chai tea leaves
- ½ teaspoon brown mica
- ½ teaspoon copper mica
- ½ teaspoon gold mica

EQUIPMENT

- Soap mold
- 2 cardboard pieces that fit tightly, lengthwise, inside the mold
- 3 large measuring cups
- Soap helper

Makes 2 pounds (907 g)

1. Make the lye solution: Add the lye to the frozen chai tea cubes as you would with any other frozen liquid (see page 105).

2. Set up the loaf mold with the cardboard inserts.

3. In the measuring cups, disperse each mica in 1 to 2 tablespoons (15 to 30 ml) melted soap oils.

4. Divide the soap batch into the three containers with the mica and mix to blend well.

5. Blend half the tea leaves into the brown soap portion and the other half into the copper portion.

6. With a soap helper, slowly pour all three portions separately into the three sections of the mold. Let the soap sit and thicken for a few minutes.

7. Slowly remove the cardboard dividers (A).

8. With a chopstick or spatula, create a mantra swirl by making figure eights through to the bottom of the soap (B).

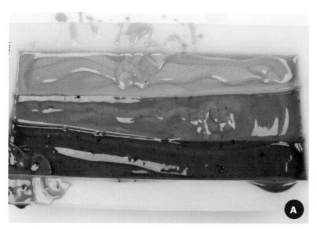

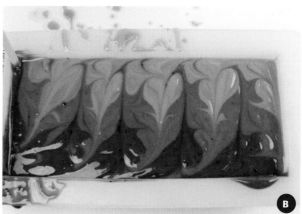

GREEN TEA LAYERED SOAP

This basic soap (use a recipe of your choosing) uses brewed green tea as a substitute for the water and adds mica and the tea leaves for color and exfoliation. (The finished soap is shown opposite, top right.)

1. Make the lye solution: Add the lye to the frozen tea cubes as you would with any other frozen liquid (see page 105).

2. In separate containers, disperse the mica and tea leaves each in 1 tablespoon (15 ml) melted soap oils.

3. Blend the fragrance oil and tea leaves into the soap and separate the batch into two parts.

4. Add the yellow mica to one portion of the soap.

5. Pour the portion of uncolored soap into the mold.

6. Pour the second colored layer into the mold, pouring over a spatula to disperse it lightly and not disturb the first layer.

INGREDIENTS
- Double-strength brewed green tea (in an equal amount to replace the water), frozen into cubes
- 1 tablespoon (14 g) brewed tea leaves per 1 lb (454 g) of soap
- ½ teaspoon yellow mica per 1 lb (454 g) of soap (you'll only use this on the top layer of soap)

EQUIPMENT
- 2 small containers
- Soap mold

Yield: Varies

Food Additives in Soap

There are other food ingredients you can add to your soap recipes that, in addition to whatever qualities they may retain after saponification, are just interesting.

When adding food to soap recipes, remember:

- Blend them in well. (No chunks!) If you leave chunks of fruit or other additives in the soap, they are likely to turn rancid or moldy, or both. Make sure the additive is completely blended into the soap.
- Generally, keep the additives to no more than 5 or 6 percent of the soap's total weight—or 1 ounce (28 g) per 1 pound (454 g) of soap.
- Consider whether you really want this ingredient in your soap. Experiment and have fun, but just because you can add it to your soap, doesn't mean you should.

Some popular foods that can be puréed and added to soap include

- Applesauce
- Avocado (especially great paired with avocado oil)
- Basil
- Carrots
- Cucumber
- Lettuce
- Peanut butter or other nut butters
- Prickly pear cactus
- Pumpkin
- Strawberries
- Tomatoes (works both as a purée or dried and ground)

Cucumber Purée Soap (left) and Pumpkin Purée Swirled Soap (right).

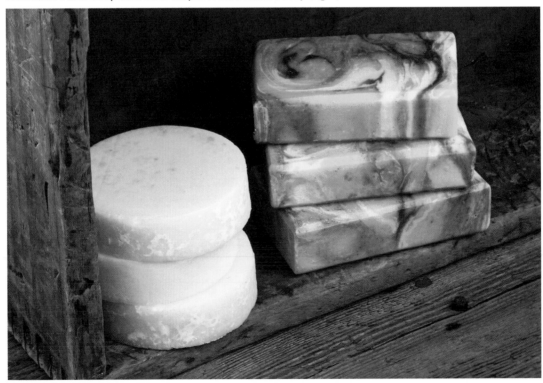

CUCUMBER PURÉE SOAP

Though it contains more than 95 percent water, the cucumber purée adds some antioxidants and fatty acids. It also adds a lovely natural pastel yellow-green color. This recipe substitutes purée for half the lye-water using the milk-in-oils method (see page 106), just with cucumber purée, not milk.

Start with a basic soap recipe of your choosing and follow standard soap-making procedures for this recipe.

INGREDIENTS
- 1 medium cucumber, peeled, peel reserved

EQUIPMENT
- Blender
- Soap molds

Yield: Varies

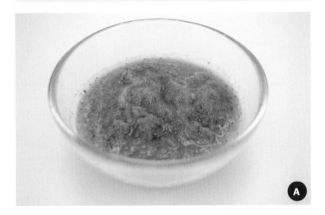

1 In a blender, finely purée the cucumber. Weigh the purée and add distilled water (or subtract purée) so it equals half the amount of water in the recipe.

2 In a blender, purée the reserved cucumber peel. Add it to the purée (A). (Don't count the peel as part of the water.)

3 Make the lye solution with the remaining water. If the lye doesn't fully dissolve, add a bit of water, 1 tablespoon (15 ml) at a time, until it fully dissolves.

4 Add the lye solution to the oils and stir to combine.

5 Blend the soap to light trace and add the fragrance or essential oil.

6 Add the cucumber and peel purées to the soap batter (B).

7 Pour the soap into the molds (C).

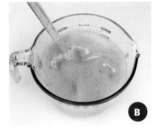
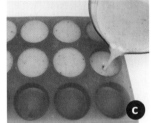

PUMPKIN PURÉE SWIRLED SOAP

Pumpkin, whether canned or freshly puréed, has long been a popular additive to soap. It contributes vitamins and a lovely natural orange color, which can be used to color the whole batch of soap, or just a portion. This recipe uses the pumpkin in the whole batch, but colors two portions of it with brown and white for an In-the-Pot Swirl (see page 90).

Start with a basic soap recipe of your choosing and follow standard soap making procedures for this recipe.

INGREDIENTS
- 2 ounces (56.5 g) canned pumpkin
- ½ teaspoon titanium dioxide
- ½ teaspoon ground cinnamon

EQUIPMENT
- 2 large measuring cups
- Soap mold

Yield: Varies

1 In the measuring cups, whisk the titanium dioxide in 1, and the cinnamon in the other, each with 1 to 2 tablespoons (15 to 30 ml) soap oils.

2 Add the lye solution to the oils and blend to light trace.

3 Mix in the pumpkin purée. Separate half the batch and divide it evenly between the two containers. Blend in the color.

4 Pour the colored soap back into opposite corners of the soap pot—one at top and bottom, one at left and right.

5 Swirl the soap with a chopstick or spatula and pour it into the mold.

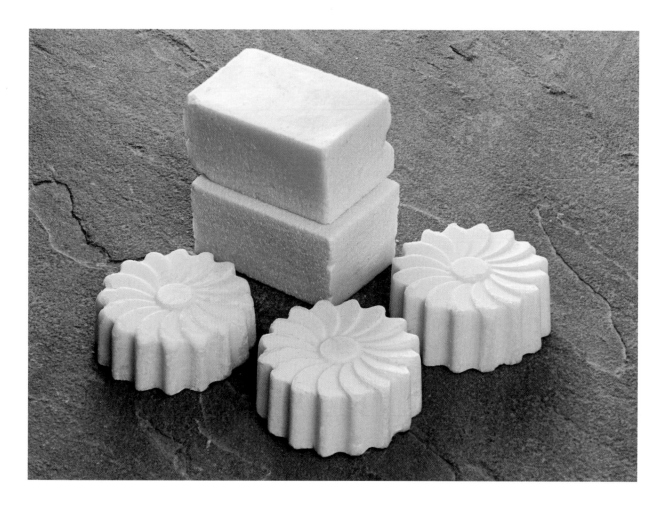

Adding Salt to Soap

Adding more than just a bit of salt to a batch of soap (to increase its hardness) creates a "salt bar," which is a wonderful combination of natural soap and bath salt. Adding it to the soap at trace leaves the salt intact so it is gently exfoliating and has the minerals and detoxifying qualities that salts in a bath would have. The salt dampens the lather considerably, so the recipe is adjusted to contain up to 80 percent coconut oil and a higher superfat percentage. The result is a rock-hard, heavy bar of soap that produces a milky, lotion-like lather that makes your skin feel wonderful.

What Sort of Salts Can I Use in My Salt Bars?

There are many varieties of salt available today, but for salt soap bars, stick with sea salt or regular table salt. Don't use Epsom or Dead Sea salts as they contain too much magnesium and other minerals that will attract water from the air and turn your soap into a mushy mess.

INGREDIENTS

- 19.5 ounces (553 g) coconut oil (75 percent)
- 2.6 ounces (74 g) lard (10 percent)
- 2.6 ounces (74 g) sunflower oil (10 percent)
- 1.3 ounces (37 g) castor oil (5 percent)

- 4 ounces (113 g) lye (about 8 percent superfat)
- 8.5 ounces (241 g) water
- 1 ounce (28 g) fragrance oil or essential oil blend
- 19.5 ounces (553 g) table salt

EQUIPMENT

- Individual cavity soap molds (see Note below)

Makes a bit more than 3.5 pounds (1.6 kg) depending on how much salt you add.

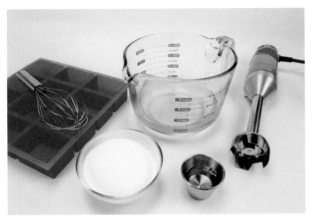

Ingredients and equipment for basic salt soap bar.

BASIC SALT BARS

For the most salt effect, you can add salt up to 100 percent of the weight of the soap oils (which, for this batch, would be 26 ounces or 737 g of salt), but the bars tend to be a bit crumbly and the lather is really dampened. I have gone as low as 50 percent of the weight of the oil, but prefer about 75 percent as a good balance between saltiness and lather.

Because the salt dampens the lather, for this recipe, start with a recipe very high in coconut oil.

1 Make a standard batch of soap using the ingredients preceding.

2 Bring the soap to light trace and add the fragrance oil.

3 Stir the salt into the soap batter, mixing it evenly (A).

4 With the addition of the salt, the soap batter will be thick. You may need to use a combination of pouring, scooping, and spreading to get the soap into the molds (B).

5 Even though the soap will be hard enough in a few hours to unmold, let it sit in the molds for 24 hours.

Note: You can use a loaf mold for salt soap, but it hardens incredibly quickly and is often difficult to slice without crumbling the bars.

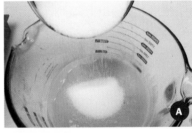

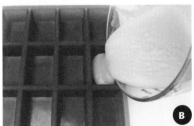

SALT SOAP VARIATION: *SOLESEIFE* OR BRINE SOAP

Traditional salt soap bars add the salt at trace, but *soleseife* soap dissolves the salt in the water before the lye is added. With the salt dissolved, the soap doesn't have the grainy, crumbly texture that regular salt bars have, but still has all the benefits of the salt—creating a rock-hard, dense-lather, long-lasting soap. This technique makes a hard, but very fine soap, so it is very well suited for intricate individual molds.

Though the lather is dampened some by the salt, it is not decreased as much as in regular salt bars, so you can use this technique with standard soap recipes. For this recipe, I used the Palm Free recipe (page 87), which has 30 percent coconut oil in it. For more lather, increase the coconut oil ratio. (Be sure to run the new recipe through a lye calculator!)

1 Add the salt to the water and stir until fully dissolved.

2 Add the lye to the saltwater and, again, stir until fully dissolved. The lye water will turn milky white (A).

3 Add the lye-saltwater solution to the oils and blend to light trace.

4 Add the fragrance oil.

5 Pour the soap into individual cavity molds. The soap should be hard enough to unmold in 8 to 10 hours.

Note: To calculate the amount of salt needed, multiply the amount of water in the recipe by 25 percent of the weight of the water in salt to dissolve. While in traditional salt bars you can add up to 100 percent of the weight of the oils in salt, with *soleseife*, the water will only allow about 25 percent of its weight in salt to dissolve.

INGREDIENTS
- Salt, an amount equal to 25 percent of the water weight in the recipe (see Note)

EQUIPMENT
- Basic soap-making equipment (see page 14)

Makes 33.5 ounces (950 g)

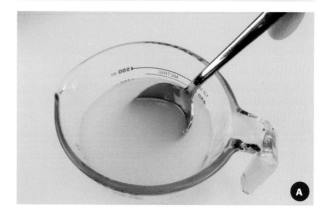

More Cold Process Soap Recipes

Between colors, scents, additives, molds, and other soap-making techniques, the variations in soaps you can create are limitless. The recipes that follow have been collected to give some examples of types and styles of soap. The ingredients and techniques are interchangeable, however. Use these recipes as starting points to create your own custom soaps.

Keeping It Simple

Often, as soap makers, we get so caught up in intricate swirls, complex scent blends, and innovative techniques. These simple, yet elegant, soaps use just one color and one scent to create a soap that can be just as wonderful as your wildest creation.

To make these soaps, start with a soap recipe of your choosing and add:

Simple Lavender

- Lavender essential oil
- Blue or purple mica or liquid colorant

Simple Grapefruit

- Grapefruit essential oil
- Red or pink mica or liquid colorant

Simple Lemon

- Lemon essential oil, or a blend of 85 percent lemon and 15 percent *litsea cubeba* (which helps anchor the lemon a bit better)
- Yellow mica or liquid colorant

Simple Mint

- Spearmint essential oil (use sparingly, mint essential oils are strong!)
- Green mica or liquid colorant

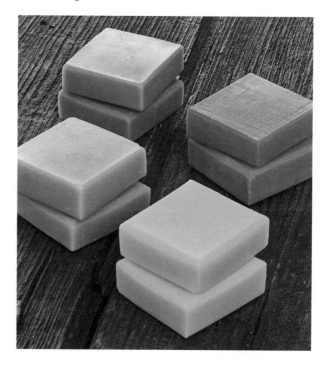

Frugal versus Luxury: Contrasting Soap Recipes

One of the following soaps is made with inexpensive ingredients from the grocery store, and one is made with 20 percent luxury butters. The soap with butter has a bit heavier and creamier lather, but both recipes make great soap!

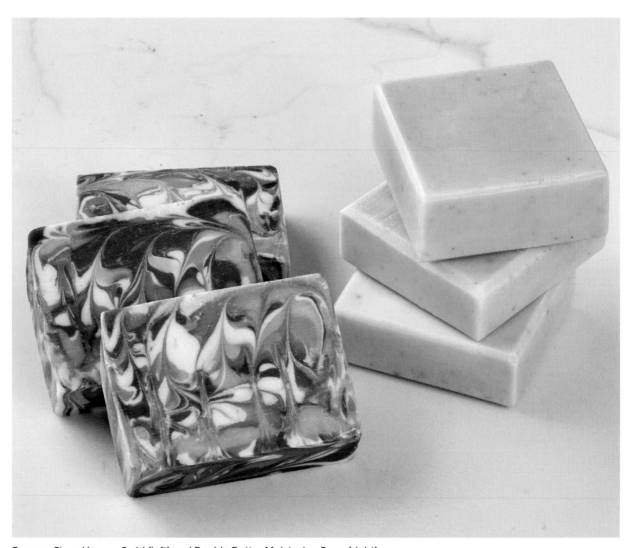

Grocery Store Hanger Swirl (left) and Double Butter Moisturing Soap (right).

DOUBLE BUTTER MOISTURIZING SOAP

INGREDIENTS

- ½ teaspoon gold mica
- ½ teaspoon copper mica
- 2.6 ounces (74 g) shea butter (10 percent)
- 2.6 ounces (74 g) cocoa butter (10 percent)
- 7.8 ounces (221 g) coconut oil (30 percent)
- 7.8 ounces (221 g) olive oil (30 percent)
- 2.6 ounces (74 g) sunflower oil (10 percent)
- 2.6 ounces (74 g) rice bran oil (10 percent)
- 3.7 ounces (105 g) lye
- 7.4 ounces (209.8 g) water

EQUIPMENT

- 2 large measuring cups
- Soap mold(s)

Makes about 2.5 pounds (1.1 kg)

1 In the measuring cups, blend each mica with 1 to 2 tablespoons (15 to 30 ml) melted soap oils.

2 Make the fresh soap with the ingredients listed. Divide the batch in two. Divide 1 batch (half the soap recipe) between the 2 containers with the micas.

3 Doing an In-the-Pot Swirl (see page 90), pour the colored soap back into the soap pot.

4 Pour the soap into the mold(s).

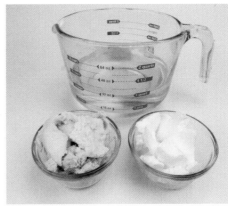

Shea butter (left) and cocoa butter (right).

GROCERY STORE HANGER SWIRL

To make this soap, use a simple recipe such as the Grocery Store (page 87).

INGREDIENTS

- ½ teaspoon green mica
- ½ teaspoon red mica
- ½ teaspoon gold mica
- ½ teaspoon titanium dioxide

EQUIPMENT

- 4 large measuring cups
- Hanger swirl tool
- Chopstick

Makes about 2 pounds (907 g)

1 In the measuring cups, blend each mica and the titanium dioxide with 1 to 2 tablespoons (15 to 30 ml) melted soap oils.

2 Make the fresh soap and divide the batch among the measuring cups and mix to blend the colorants.

3 Layer the soap colors in the loaf mold a bit at a time, one after the other.

4 Use a hanger swirl tool in an up-and-down pattern (see page 94) to swirl the soap.

5 Using a chopstick, swirl the top 0.5 inch (1 cm) of the soap.

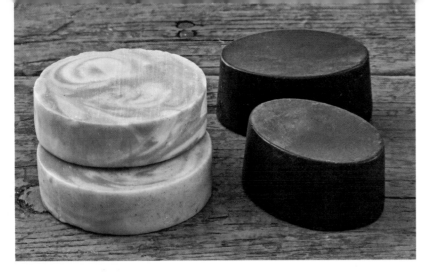

Detoxifying Spa Soaps

These two soaps use ingredients known for their absorbent and detoxifying qualities—activated charcoal and earth clays.

TEA TREE AND CHARCOAL SOAP

To make this soap, shown above right, start with a basic soap recipe, such as the Basic (page 86).

INGREDIENTS

- 2 teaspoons activated charcoal per 1 lb (454 g) of soap oils
- Essential oil blend, consisting of
  - 50 percent tea tree essential oil
  - 35 percent lavender essential oil
  - 15 percent patchouli essential oil

EQUIPMENT

- Soap.molds

Makes 2 pounds (907 g)

1 Mix the charcoal into 2 tablespoons (30 ml) melted soap oils.

2 Make the fresh soap batch as normal, adding the charcoal and essential oil blend at trace.

3 Pour the soap into the molds.

TRIPLE CLAY SWIRLED SOAP

Start with a slow-moving soap recipe, such as the Slow Mover (page 87), shown above left.

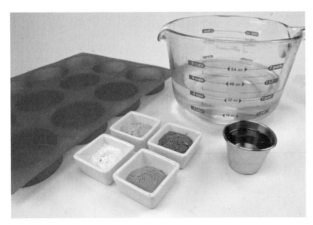

INGREDIENTS

- ½ teaspoon rhassoul clay
- ½ teaspoon green sea clay
- ½ teaspoon red Moroccan clay
- 1 teaspoon titanium dioxide
- 1 ounce (28 g) essential oil blend of choice

EQUIPMENT

- 3 large measuring cups
- Distilled water
- Ramekin
- Chopstick or spatula
- Soap molds
- Rubbing alcohol

Make 2 pounds (907 g)

Clays, oils, and mold for Triple Clay Swirled Soap. Clockwise from upper left: green clay, red clay, rhassoul clay, and titanium dioxide.

1. In the measuring cups, mix the rhassoul, green sea, and red Moroccan clays each with 3 tablespoons (45 ml) distilled water. (Clay absorbs water, so this helps them not accelerate the trace in your soap batch.)

2. In a ramekin, mix the titanium dioxide with 2 tablespoons (40 ml) water as well.

3. Make the fresh soap batch as normal, adding the essential oil blend to the oils before adding the lye. Blend the soap to light trace.

4. Divide half the batch among the three containers.

5. Add the titanium dioxide to the soap pot and blend.

6. Using an In-the-Pot Swirl (page 90), pour one color in each corner of a triangle—top, bottom right, and bottom left (A).

7. Using a chopstick or spatula, swirl the soap in the pot in a circular/spiral pattern (B).

8. Pour the soap into the molds.

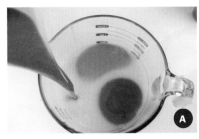

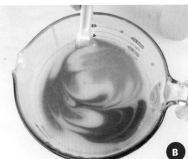

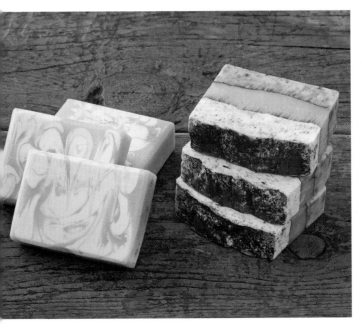

NATURAL PAPRIKA SWIRL

To make this soap, shown far left, start with a basic soap recipe, such as the Basic (page 86), with 50 percent of the olive oil substituted with a paprika-infused oil (see page 81).

INGREDIENTS
- ½ teaspoon titanium dioxide

EQUIPMENT
- Soap mold
- Hanger swirl tool (see page 95)

Makes 2 pounds (907 g)

1. Mix the titanium dioxide with 2 tablespoons (30 ml) melted soap oils.

2. Make the soap batch as normal, substituting the paprika-infused oil for 50 percent of the olive oil in your recipe, fragrance oil at a very light trace.

3. Separate the batch into 2 parts and mix 1 part with the titanium dioxide.

4. Pour the uncolored soap into the mold.

5. From a height of 4 to 5 inches (10 to 13 cm) drizzle the whitened soap into the mold. (The height allows the soap to penetrate further into the soap.)

6. Using a hanger swirl tool, swirl the soap with the Curls and Swirls pattern (see page 95).

CHAMOMILE AND CALENDULA

This three-layer soap, shown on page 121, bottom right, uses natural ground calendula flowers and chamomile, along with a mica line to make a soap that is both elegant and natural.

To make this soap, start with a slow-moving recipe, such as the Slow Mover (page 87).

INGREDIENTS

- 2 tablespoons (4 g) ground chamomile flowers
- 1 tablespoon (2 g) chopped or torn calendula flowers
- ½ teaspoon yellow mica
- ½ teaspoon titanium dioxide
- 1 ounce (28 g) fragrance oil or essential oil
- About 1 teaspoon burgundy mica

EQUIPMENT

- 3 large measuring cups
- Mesh tea strainer

Make 2 pounds (907 g)

1 In the measuring cups, mix 2 tablespoons of the melted oils with: a. half of the chamomile, b. the calendula flowers and yellow mica, and c. half of the chamomile and the titanium dioxide.

2 Spoon the burgundy mica into the tea strainer.

3 Make the fresh soap batch as normal, adding the fragrance oil at light trace.

4 Divide the batch among the three containers. Stir to blend.

5 Pour the chamomile only into the mold.

6 Tapping the tea strainer closely over the soap, lightly coat the first layer with a layer of mica. When you've covered most of the soap, move about 6 inches (15 cm) away from the soap, close your eyes, and gently blow on the soap. This will evenly disperse the mica.

7 Pouring over a spatula, gently pour the calendula and yellow mica portion onto the first layer, being careful not to disturb the mica or the first layer.

8 Repeat step 6 with the mica.

9 Again, pouring over a spatula, pour the chamomile and titanium dioxide portion over the second layer.

10 Sprinkle a bit more mica on top of the soap.

WILDFLOWER SHREDS SOAP

This is a favorite of Maggie Hanus of A Wild Soap Bar in Manor, Texas. Maggie uses only wild and organic herbs and 100 percent-certified organic vegetable oils. She also doesn't like to waste any scraps, so she shreds and incorporates them into her Wildflower Soap. The shreds have a potpourri and floral scent blend.

INGREDIENTS

- See Basic Method for Making Cold Process Soap (page 78) for the basic ingredients list. You'll need to adjust the recipe to accommodate the amount of shredded soap scraps you plan to include.

EQUIPMENT

- Basic soap making equipment (see page 14)
- Grater or knife (for shredding or cutting the soap)
- Soap mold

Yield: Varies

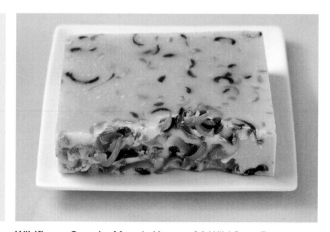

Wildflower Soap by Maggie Hanus of A Wild Soap Bar.

1 Calculate the ratio of shreds to the amount of fresh soap you want in your batch. One-third shreds to two-thirds fresh soap is typical.

2 Weigh the appropriate amount of soap to use for shreds in your batch.

3 Shred your soap scraps or cut them into small chunks. Set aside.

4 Adjust your soap recipe so the amount of shreds plus the amount of fresh soap will equal the total amount of soap you want to make.

5 Mix your new batch of soap and bring it to a light trace.

6 Add the appropriate amount of scent to the fresh soap.

7 Set aside a small amount of the shreds. Stir the remaining shreds into the fresh soap and pour the mixture into the mold.

8 Sprinkle the reserved shreds evenly over the top of the soap. Push them down lightly so they will stick in the fresh soap mixture.

LAYERED SHREDS SOAP

This is another recipe where you can use up odds and ends of other bars you've made. Instead of mixing shreds into the whole bar, as with the Wildflower Soap (see opposite page), this recipe layers assorted colors and types of shreds separately. Though this recipe calls for three layers of shreds and a top layer of fresh soap, you can create your own variation.

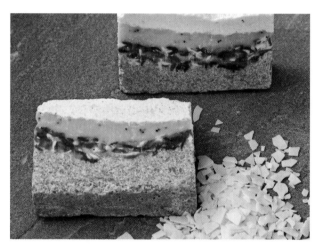

Layered Shreds Soap.

INGREDIENTS

- See Basic Method for Making Cold Process Soap (page 78) for the basic ingredients list. You'll need to adjust the recipe to accommodate the number and amount of shredded soap scraps you plan to include.
- ½ teaspoon (2 g) titanium dioxide per 1 lb (454 g) of fresh soap (to create a white base)

EQUIPMENT

- Basic soap-making equipment (see page 14)
- Grater or knife (for shredding or cutting the soap)

Yield: Varies

1 Calculate the ratio of shreds to the amount of fresh soap you want in your batch. The soap shown in the photo has four layers—three layers of shreds and one layer of fresh soap—so I only needed to make one third of the basic cold process soap recipe. I used some of that batch to bind the shreds of each layer together, and the rest as the top layer.

- Bottom layer: goat's milk/oatmeal shreds
- Third layer: blue and white swirled shreds
- Second layer: lemon–poppy seed shreds
- Top layer: fresh soap with titanium dioxide added

2 Make enough fresh soap to equal about one third of the total batch.

3 Add just enough fresh soap to each portion of shreds to make the shreds stick together.

4 Layer each shred mixture separately by pouring or scooping it into the mold.

5 Add the titanium dioxide to the remaining fresh soap and pour it into the mold as the top layer.

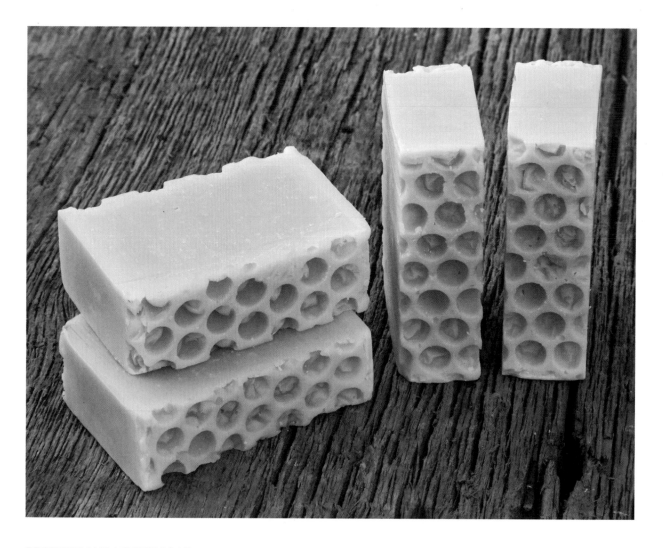

BEESWAX AND HONEY SOAP

Some soap recipe ingredients have direct effects on the soap. Honey, for example, helps increase the lather and imparts a golden color to the soap. Beeswax contributes less to the soap, adding only some hardness. But the two together, along with this bubble wrap technique, evoke a warm, natural, sweet-smelling, buzzing honeycomb.

INGREDIENTS

- 6.2 ounces (175.76 g) water
- 2 teaspoons honey
- 3 ounces (88 g) lye
- 0.5 ounce (14 g) beeswax (2 percent)
- 8.8 ounces (249.5 g) olive oil (40 percent)
- 6.6 ounces (187 g) coconut oil (30 percent)
- 3 ounces (82 g) sunflower oil (13 percent)
- 2.2 ounces (62 g) cocoa butter (10 percent)
- 1 ounce (31 g) castor oil (5 percent)
- 1 ounce (28 g) fragrance oil or essential oil

EQUIPMENT

- Bubble wrap
- Basic soap-making equipment (see page 14)
- Soap mold

Makes 2 pounds (907 g)

1 Cut two pieces of bubble wrap to fit the length and width of the soap mold. Place one piece on the bottom of the mold (A).

2 Take 3 tablespoons (45 ml) of the water for your lye solution and mix it with the honey (B).

3 Make the lye solution with the remaining water.

4 Melt the beeswax in a separate container. It must reach about 145° (63°C) to melt, much hotter than the other oils.

5 Melt the soap oils to at least 120°F (49°C).

6 Add the melted beeswax to the soap oils and stir. If any beeswax solidifies and won't blend into the oils, heat the oils a bit more until it does (C).

7 Blend the water–honey mix into the soap oils.

8 Add the fragrance oil.

9 Add the lye solution to the oils and blend to light trace.

10 Pour the soap batter into the mold (D).

11 Place the second piece of bubble wrap on top of the soap and gently press it into the soap (E).

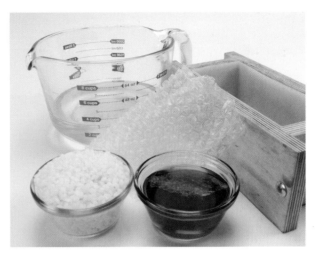

Beeswax, honey, and bubble wrap for Beeswax and Honey Soap.

12 Cover and insulate the soap well. It will go through a very hot gel stage (F).

13 Let it sit overnight and slice it the next day. Let it cure for 3 to 4 weeks.

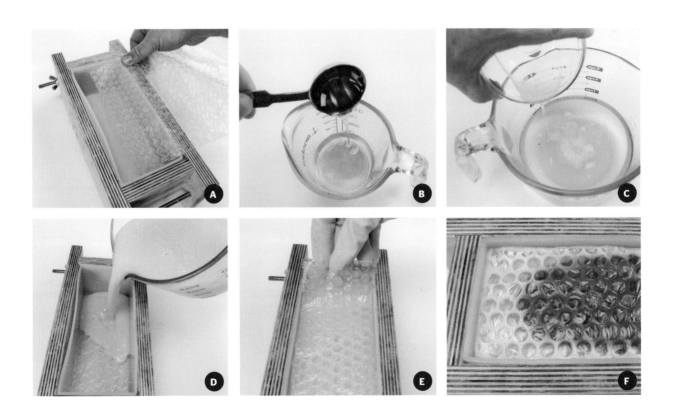

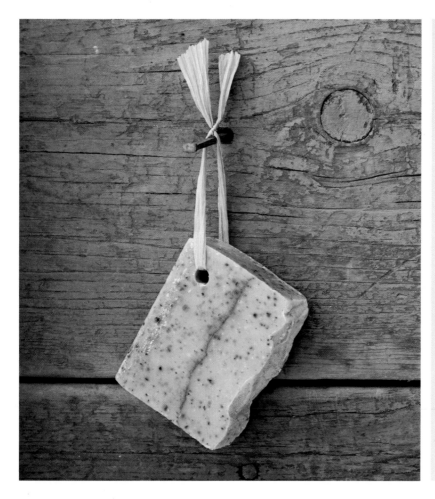

IINGREDIENTS

- See Basic Method for Making Cold Process Soap (page 78) for the basic ingredients list.
- About 1 tablespoon (28 g) used/brewed coffee grounds (1.5 teaspoons or 7.5 g per 1 lb [454 g] of soap)
- ¼ to ½ teaspoon dark-colored mica

EQUIPMENT

- Basic soap making equipment (see page 14)
- Soap mold
- Tea strainer

Makes 2 pounds (907 g) soap or about eight (4-ounce or 113 g) bars

COFFEE SOAP WITH MICA LINE

Mixing used coffee grounds into a batch of cold process soap adds a natural exfoliant as well as rich color. This soap is also enhanced with a layer of mica colorant in the middle.

1 Make a 2 pound (907 g) batch of soap. Bring it to light trace and add your fragrance oil.

2 Add the coffee grounds and mix them into the soap. Pour half the soap batch into your mold.

3 Place the mica into the tea strainer. If you want a flat mica line, tap the mold on the counter first to level the soap. If you want a wavy line, use a spatula to stir the soap first.

4 Lightly tap the strainer over the soap in the mold. Lay down a light, uniform layer of mica—just barely enough so you can't see the soap underneath it. Close your eyes and gently blow on the mica to disperse it evenly.

5 Gently pour the second half of the soap into the mold.

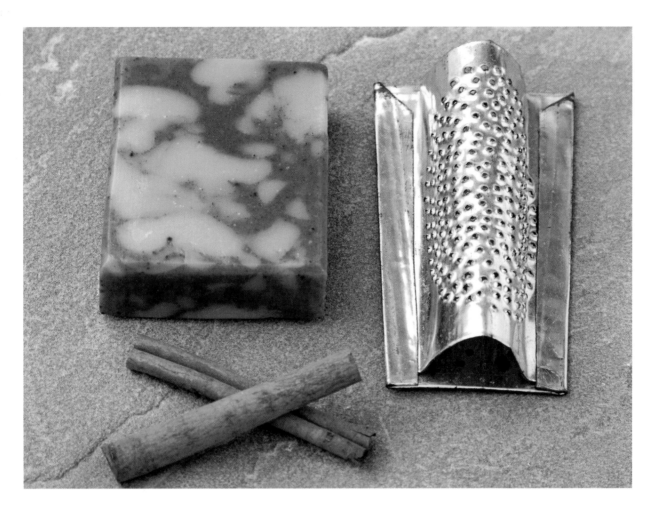

CINNAMON SWIRL SOAP

For this soap, start with a slow-moving soap recipe, scaled to 2 pounds (908 g) such as the Slow Mover (page 87).

INGREDIENTS

- ½ teaspoon ground cinnamon
- ½ teaspoon tsp red or brown oxide, or gold mica, or a combination of all three
- 1 ounce (28 g) fragrance oil or essential oil

EQUIPMENT

- 2 large measuring cups
- Hanger swirl tool
- Soap mold

Makes 2 pounds (907 g)

1 In the two measuring cups, mix the cinnamon (in one) and oxide or mica (in the other) with 1 to 2 tablespoons (15 to 30 ml) melted soap oils.

2 Make the fresh soap batch as normal, adding the fragrance oil at light trace.

3 Separate half the soap batch and divide it between the cinnamon and mica measuring cups. Stir to blend.

4 Pour the colored soaps back into the soap pot and gently swirl.

5 Pour the soap into the mold.

DOUBLE OMBRÉ SOAP WITH ALKANET

This advanced soap recipe uses natural alkanet color in a layered ombré effect, getting lighter from the bottom up. Titanium dioxide is gradually added from the bottom up to enhance the effect.

Start with slow-moving recipe such as the Slow Mover (page 87; scaled to 3 pounds [1.4 kg]) and follow standard soap-making procedures for this recipe.

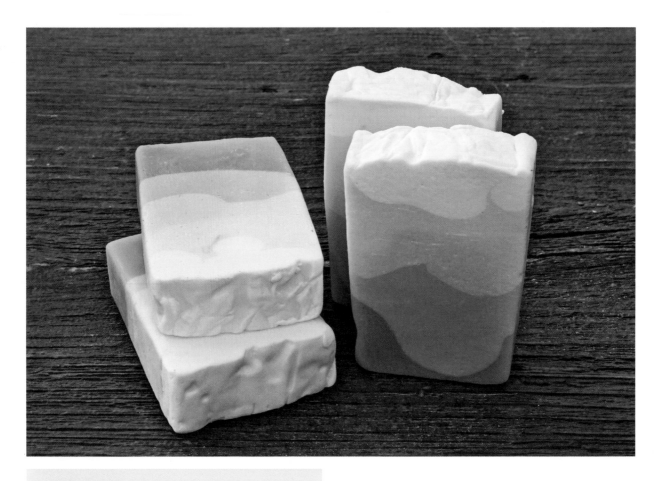

INGREDIENTS
- 2 teaspoons titanium dioxide
- 10 tablespoons (150 ml) previously made alkanet-infused olive oil (see page 81)
- 1.3 ounces (37 g) fragrance oil or essential oil

EQUIPMENT
- 3 large measuring cups
- 5 medium-size containers
- Soap mold
- Rubbing alcohol

Makes 3 pounds (1.36 kg)

1 Measure the olive oil needed for your recipe and place it in a measuring cup.

2 Transfer 10 tablespoons (150 ml) of this base olive oil amount into a separate container.

3 Mix the titanium dioxide into these 10 tablespoons (150 ml) of olive oil.

4 Measure 10 tablespoons (150 ml) more of the base olive oil and pour it back into the olive oil bottle.

5 Put the alkanet-infused olive oil into a measuring cup.

6 Set up five containers (A) and in each put

- Into container 1: 4 tablespoons (60 ml) alkanet oil

- Into container 2: 3 tablespoons (45 ml) alkanet oil plus 1 tablespoon (15 ml) titanium dioxide oil
- Into container 3: 2 tablespoons (30 ml) alkanet oil plus 2 tablespoons (30 ml) titanium oxide oil
- Into container 4: 1 tablespoon (15 ml) alkanet oil plus 3 tablespoons (45 ml) titanium oxide oil
- Into container 5: 4 tablespoons (60 ml) titanium oxide oil

7 Measure and prepare the remaining soap recipe ingredients (B).

8 Mix the lye with the oils and bring to light trace.

9 Evenly divide the soap among the 5 containers. Mix to blend (C).

10 Starting with the darkest all-alkanet soap, pour the soap into the mold (D).

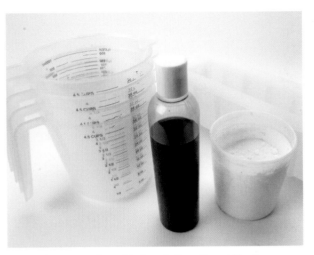

Measuring cups, alkanet-infused olive oil, and titanium dioxide for Double Ombre Soap.

11 Pouring over a spatula, pour the next-darkest color of soap into the mold (E).

12 Repeat until you've poured the final all-white layer into the mold (F).

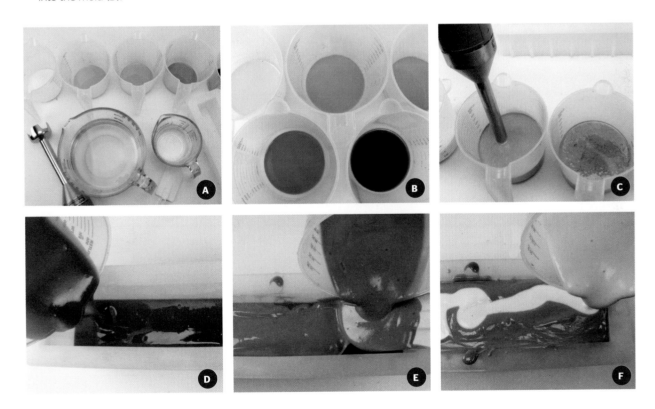

Cold Process Companion Bath and Body Products

Once you've set up a collection of equipment, fragrances, oils, and additives, there are several other bath and body products you can make with the same, or just a few extra, ingredients.

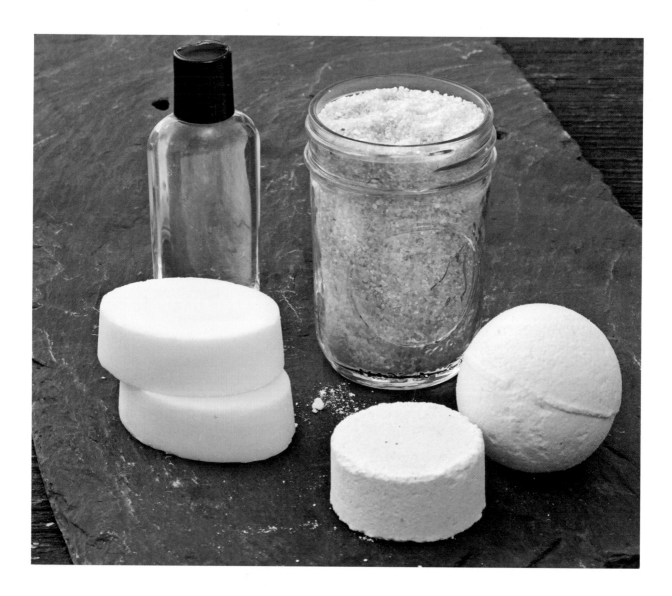

Bath Salts

Although it seems that the simple bath is an old-fashioned custom, adding a specially formulated bath salt can transform a boring bath into a wonderful soak. Starting with plain salt, a variety of other salts can be added:

- Epsom salts: high in magnesium, relaxing, and soothing to muscles
- Dead Sea salts: full of beneficial trace minerals
- Baking soda: detoxifying, soothing, and cleansing

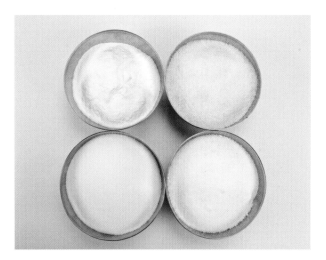

Other ingredients can be added as well. Oatmeal and milk powders can be soothing and moisturizing to the skin. Flower petals contribute a bit of scent and luxury floating in the bath. Consider

- Chamomile flowers
- Ground oatmeal
- Lavender buds
- Milk powder
- Rose petals

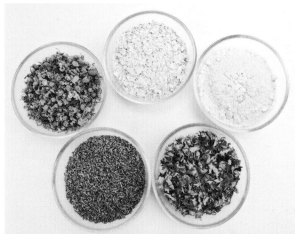

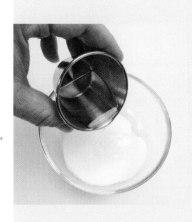 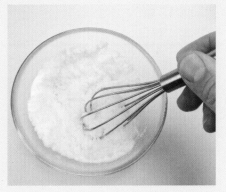

Using Dendritic Salt

Dendritic salt is a type of salt that has a crystalline structure that binds better to fragrance oils. Using about 5 percent dendritic salt in any recipe will help the salts retain their fragrance better. When making the salt blend, measure the dendritic salt and stir the fragrance oil directly into it. Add the mixture to the remaining ingredients.

SIMPLE MILK BATH

INGREDIENTS

- 2 cups (250 g) powdered milk
- 1 cup (249 g) Epsom salts
- 1 cup (288 g) sea salt
- 0.5 cup (110.5 g) baking soda
- 0.5 ounce (14 g) fragrance oil or essential oil

Makes 4.5 cups (911.5 g)

OATMEAL BATH SALTS

INGREDIENTS

- 1 cup (80 g) finely ground oatmeal
- 1 cup (288 g) sea salt
- 1 cup (249 g) Epsom salt
- 0.25 ounce (7 g) fragrance oil or essential oil

Makes 3 cups (617 g)

BASIC BATH SALTS

INGREDIENTS

- 3 cups (705 ml) Epsom salt
- 2 cups (470 ml) sea salt
- 1 cup (221 g) baking soda
- 0.5 ounce (14 g) fragrance oil or essential oil

Makes 6 cups (1.55 kg)

HERBAL BATH TEA

INGREDIENTS

- 2 cups (470 ml) blended bath salts
- 0.25 cup (9 g) lavender buds
- 0.25 cup (8 g) chamomile flowers
- 0.25 ounce (7 g) fragrance oil or essential oil

Makes 2.5 cups (537 g)

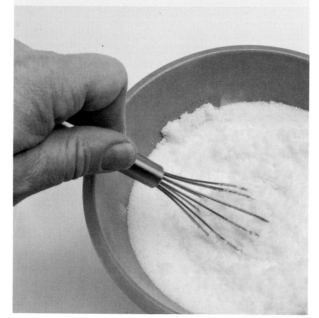

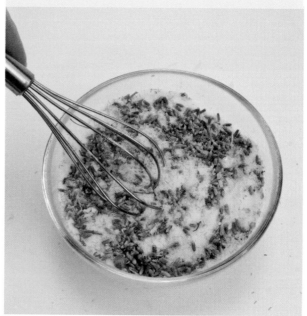

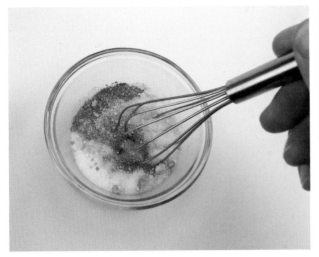

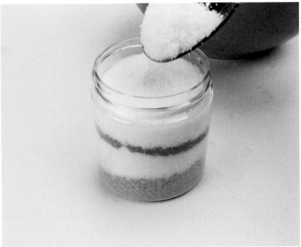

Adding Color to Bath Salts

Most colorants used for soap can also be used in bath salts. Sprinkle a bit of mica into the salt and stir to mix, or add a couple drops of liquid colorant. With their larger crystalline structure, Epsom salts hold the color better.

Layered Bath Salts

Layer white and colored bath salts in the same jar. Leave the layers as they are or use a chopstick to create designs in the layers.

Water-Dispersible Bath Oils

Simple bath oils can be made by combining any of the lighter soap making oils, such as jojoba, grape seed, almond, or rice bran, and fragrance or essential oils. But in a bath, the oils float on top of the water and leave a ring around the tub. Adding an emulsifier, such as polysorbate 80, helps the oils disperse through-out the bath and rinse off more easily.

INGREDIENTS

- 0.2 ounce (5.6 g) fragrance or essential oil (5 percent)
- 0.8 ounce (22.7 g) polysorbate 80 (20 percent)
- 3 ounces (85 g) light oil (75 percent)

EQUIPMENT

- Plastic bottle (colored or clear) with a lid

Makes 4 ounces

1 Pour the fragrance or essential oil into the bottle.

2 Add the polysorbate 80, cover the bottle, and shake well.

3 Add the light oil to the mixture. Cover and shake well.

4 Shake before each use.

Fizzy Bath Bombs

Bath bombs are a combination of bath salt and bath oil that are easy to make and wonderful in the bath. The basic formula is two parts baking soda and one part citric acid, which make the "fizz." Additional ingredients bring scent, soothing, and moisturizing.

INGREDIENTS: DRY PHASE

- 2 cups (442 g) baking soda
- 1 cup (150 g) citric acid
- 1 cup (128 g) cornstarch
- 0.5 cup (124.5 g) Epsom salt
- 0.5 cup (144 g) sea salt

INGREDIENTS: WET PHASE

- 2 tsp water
- ½ teaspoon borax or 1 teaspoon polysorbate 80
- 1 to 2 teaspoons fragrance oil or essential oil
- 2 tablespoons (30 ml) light oil, such as jojoba, grape seed, almond, or rice bran

Makes about 2 pounds (907 g) bath bombs

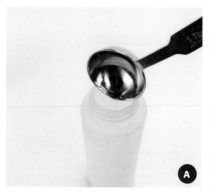 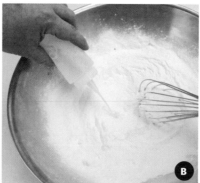 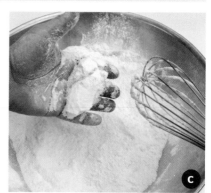

1 Into a large, wide bowl, sift together all the dry phase ingredients. Whisk to combine.

2 In a small squeeze bottle, combine the wet phase ingredients (A).

3 Squirt several drops of the liquid into the dry ingredients. It will start to fizz (B). Stir the liquid into the dry ingredients.

4 Continue to add the liquid, 1 small squirt at a time, quickly stirring the liquid into the mixture each time. As the liquid is added, the mixture will begin to feel heavy, like wet sand.

5 When all the liquid is added, grasp a handful of the mixture, squeeze it, and move it around gently in your hand. If it holds together, the mixture is ready (C).

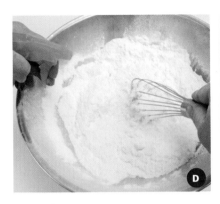
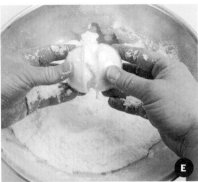
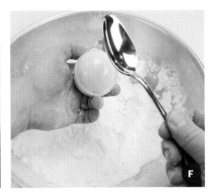

6 If it falls apart, using a spray bottle, spray a small amount of water into the mixture and stir (D). After each couple of sprays, test the mixture to see if it holds together. Go slowly. You do not want to add too much water to the mix!

7 When the mixture is ready, mold it in small cosmetic containers, small individual soap molds, or (as shown) two-part plastic balls (E). Press and compact the mixture as tightly as possible in the mold. Squeeze the mold halves together and hold for 5 to 10 seconds.

8 To unmold the bombs, tap one side with a tablespoon and gently squeeze the mold (F).

9 Cupping the bomb in your other hand, remove the other half of the mold.

10 Set the bombs aside on a paper-towel lined baking sheet to dry overnight.

11 They will be very fragile at this point and may fall apart. If this happens, just scoop the mixture back into the bowl and remold the bomb.

Adding Color and Botanicals to Bath Bombs

- A few drops of liquid colorant can be added into the wet phase, if desired. This will give a uniform pastel color to the bombs.

- Adding ½ to 1 teaspoon mica or oxide during the dry phase will give a speckled, variegated color to the bombs.

- Botanicals, such as flower petals and oatmeal, can be added during the dry phase as well, or sprinkle a few flower petals into the mold before adding the mixture to mold the botanicals onto just one side of the bomb.

Bath Bomb Variations

SHOWER BOMBS

Shower bombs are intended to add fragrance to the shower, so the skin-soothing ingredients are omitted.

Make the shower bombs as you would bath bombs (see page 134). Ice cube trays work well for molds and are an appropriate size for shower bombs.

INGREDIENTS: DRY PHASE

- 2 cups (442 g) baking soda
- 1 cup (150 g) citric acid

INGREDIENTS: WET PHASE

- 2 teaspoons water
- ½ teaspoon borax or 1 teaspoon polysorbate 80

- 1 to 2 teaspoons essential oil or fragrance oil

Makes about 1.3 pounds (590 g) shower bombs

TOILET BOMBS

The toilet bomb's fizzing action helps clean the toilet bowl while the fragrance or essential oil leaves a pleasant scent.

Make the toilet bombs as you would bath bombs (see page 134). They can be molded in a variety of sizes and stored in a jar next to the toilet.

INGREDIENTS: DRY PHASE

- 2 cups (442 g) baking soda
- 1 cup (150 g) citric acid
- 0.5 cup (204.5 g) borax

INGREDIENTS: WET PHASE

- 1 teaspoon hydrogen peroxide
- 1 teaspoon white vinegar

- 1 tablespoon (15 ml) fragrance oil or essential oil

Makes about 1.9 pounds (850 g) toilet bombs

Solid Massage/Lotion Bars

A solid massage/lotion bar is a combination of oils that are solid at room temperature, but melt when it comes in contact with skin. Most any combination of oils can be used, but you must balance between hard and liquid oils to achieve the final melting point.

INGREDIENTS

- 3 ounces (85 g) beeswax
- 3 ounces (85 g) cocoa butter
- 3 ounces (85 g) light liquid oil
- 0.25 ounce (7 g) essential oil or fragrance oil (optional)

Make 8 massage bars

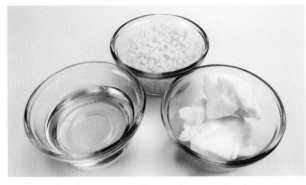

Liquid oil, left, beeswax, and cocoa butter—simple ingredients for solid massage/lotion bars.

1 Melt the oils, starting with the hardest (the beeswax) first.

2 When the beeswax is fully melted, add the cocoa butter (A) and stir to mix.

3 When the beeswax and cocoa butter are melted, add the liquid oil and stir to mix.

4 Let the oils cool to below 150° (65.5°C) before adding any fragrance oil (if using).

5 Pour the mixture into individual molds to cool and harden (B).

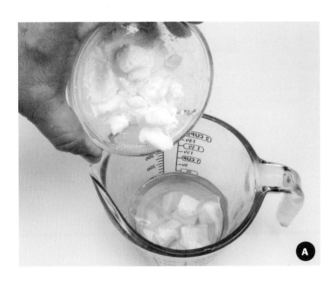

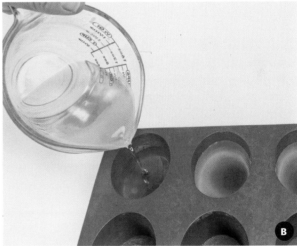

Storing Handmade Soap

Hand-milled, cold process, and hot process soaps can all be stored and packaged in the same way. All these soaps need time to cure after they're finished and unmolded. Curing is the time the soap needs for the excess water to evaporate. Although the chemical reaction may be complete, the soaps need to dry and harden. Most soap makers agree that a fully cured bar is also milder, lasts longer in the shower, and lathers better.

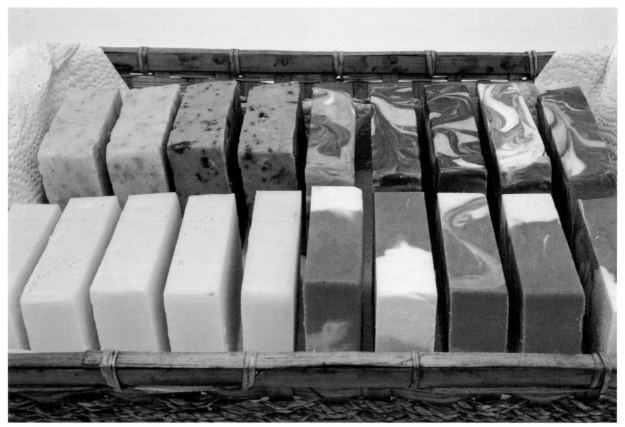

Store your soaps during and after curing in a cool, dry place in a container lined with paper towels. Cover with a light towel to keep dust from settling on them.

The key to storing your soaps and letting them cure is to give them some air and room to breathe. Line a shelf, shoebox, basket, or other container with a layer of paper towels and set the soaps on their ends with a bit of space between each bar. Set them in a cool, dry place and cover them with a light towel to keep any dust off. Most soaps will be fully cured in four to six weeks. Note that soaps containing high amounts of olive oil need longer than six weeks to cure. Castile soaps, which contain 100 percent olive oil, can take up to 6 months to harden fully.

Packaging Your Soap

Soap for personal use doesn't need to be packaged or wrapped. It is just fine sitting in a basket or on a shelf. If you want to package your soap to sell or give as gifts, there are many popular simple methods you can try.

Shrink-wrap or plastic wrap with a sticker. Wrap your soap in plastic or shrink-wrap, with the ends wrapped around the back. Place a printed sticker on the front and/or the back that identifies the soap. Some plastic and shrink-wraps allow the scent to come through. Shrink-wrap soap bands allow you to leave small openings at the ends of the soap.

Cigar band. This label can be used with or without shrink-wrap or plastic wrap. Measure the circumference of the bar of soap you want to wrap and add about 0.5 inch (1.3 cm). Cut a strip of heavy paper or card stock to that length and to a width that looks good on the bar of soap. Print the paper or card stock with graphics or text. (Keep in mind you may need to flip or otherwise adjust the position of some of the text or other elements, depending on where they appear on the label.) Cut out the label and wrap it around the soap, affixing the overlapping ends with a bit of glue. Note: If you wrap your soap before it's fully cured, it will continue to shrink as the water evaporates and the label will become loose on the bar.

Full paper wrap. Wrap your soap with a piece of decorative paper, just as you would wrap a gift. Affix a label to the front and/or the back.

Soap boxes. A number of packaging vendors offer boxes made specifically for bars of soap. Some have small cutouts on one side so the soap is visible, while others are completely enclosed. As with the full paper wrap, a label can be affixed to the box.

Specialty bags and boxes. There are a multitude of other decorative ways to package your soaps, from small, plain muslin pouches to shiny organza bags, plastic bags, boxes, and more.

Labeling Soap

Entire books have been written about the regulations for labeling handmade soaps and cosmetics for retail sale. In the United States, if it's labeled "soap," without making any cosmetic or medical claims, the key information that must be on the packaging includes:

- Ingredients
- Weight
- Maker's or manufacturer's contact information

The regulations are complex and vary from country to country, so make sure your soaps are properly labeled if you sell them.

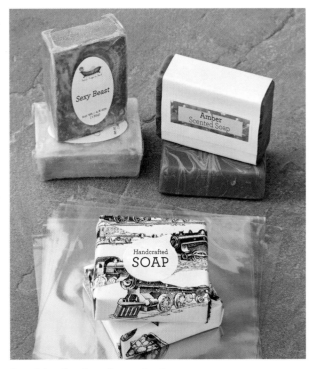

A variety of options for packaging soap.

Cold Process Soap:
Tips and Troubleshooting

Cold process soap making is a pretty reliable and straightforward process if ingredients are measured accurately and the steps are carefully followed.

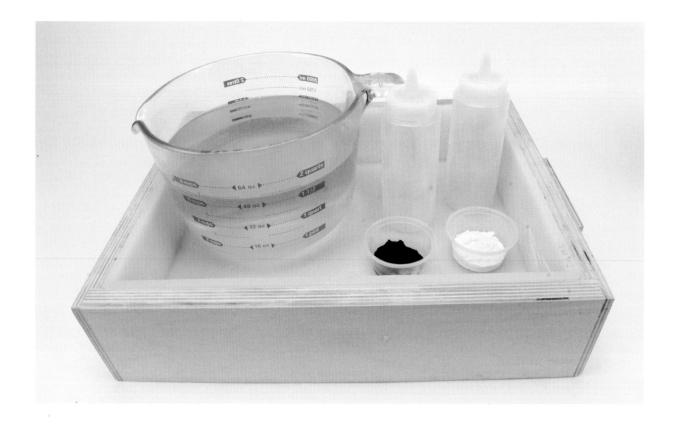

Tips for Cold Process Soap

1   Be relaxed, but work methodically. Most problems occur when an ingredient is left out or mismeasured. Being too hurried or stressed can create as many errors as being too distracted. *This is also when accidents happen.*

2   Keep a soap scrapbook or online file of soaps you want to make. They will motivate you to try new techniques and keep your love of soap making strong.

3   Never, ever, make soap without proper eye protection. I am guilty of making soap without gloves, but over all my years of soap making, I have always worn eye protection.

4   Keep a bar or two of your very first batch of soap. I have two bars of my first batch and I cherish them as much as any bars I've ever made.

Troubleshooting Cold Process Soap

Even the most experienced soap makers have a batch, now and then, that doesn't turn out quite right. It can be frustrating and even heartbreaking. Some batches can be saved. Some are better not. Most soap-batch troubles are due to a few common problems:

- Problems with measuring
- Problems with mixing
- Problems with ingredients

Problems with Measuring or Missing Ingredients

The first things to ask yourself when a batch has a problem are, "Did I leave any ingredients out? Did I measure everything correctly?" If you left an ingredient out, and you know *exactly* what ingredient it is (for example, you left out an oil), you can rebatch the soap and it will be fine (see page 26).

If you fear you have measured something incorrectly or left something out that you aren't sure of, the batch is best discarded. You are just guessing as to how to fix and properly balance it.

If you have a batch of soap that won't harden, or is hard and crumbly, there is a good chance that you mismeasured an ingredient. Soap that won't harden probably does not enough lye or has too much water in it. Soap that is hard and crumbly probably has too much lye or too much sodium lactate.

Problems with Mixing

Although immersion (stick) blenders have made mixing soap to emulsion or trace immensely easier than it used to be, sometimes, batches won't be mixed quite enough. This can lead to separation.

- Separation of the oils and lye
- Separation of some of the fragrance oil from the rest of the soap
- Separation of small amounts of lye from the rest of the soap

What to do about it? If the whole batch has separated, and you're sure you measured everything correctly, chop it up and put it in a slow cooker to rebatch (see page 26).

If there are just a few little pockets or pools of liquid that have seeped out of the soap, do a tongue test (see below) on them to see if it is oil or lye. If it is oil, leave it for a day. Often it will reabsorb into the soap. If it's lye, you'll need to rebatch the soap.

Tongue Test

You can do this simple test on either a fresh bar of cold process soap or cooked soap.

- **For cold process:** Touch the tip of your tongue to the finished soap. If you get any "zap," wait the full cure time and test again. If you still get a "zap" after 3 or 4 days, the soap is lye heavy and, unfortunately, needs to be tossed out.
- **For hot process:** Dip the back of a spoon into the soap. Let it cool and touch the tip of your tongue to the soap. If you get any "zap," it needs to cook longer. If it just tastes like soap, the cooking is done. If, as with cold process, you continue to get "zap," the soap is lye heavy and needs to be discarded.

How to Prevent Separation

With immersion blenders, this is a rare problem. It is more likely to happen when soaping at very low (less than 90°F or 32°C) temperatures. At very low temperatures, the oils start to resolidify, which looks like trace but is actually a false trace. If working at very low temperatures, mix very thoroughly and monitor the batch for separation over its first few hours in the mold. If the soap begins to separate, gently stir it in the mold. If it continues to separate, scoop the whole batch into a slow cooker and hot process it.

Problems with Ingredients

Most soap-making vendors give you useful information about ingredients, fragrance oils, or essential oils that can be troublesome, and sometimes, the ingredients will just surprise you.

Soap that gets thick very quickly in the pot (acceleration).
- This can be caused by many fragrance and essential oils. Some (such as floral and spice oils) will cause the soap to come to trace almost immediately.
- It can also be caused by recipes that are very high in hard oils and butters.
- When it gets *super* thick—almost like putty—it's called a seize, or "soap on a stick."

What to do about it? If this happens, just do your best to scoop the soap into a mold and spread it into shape. The problem should just be aesthetic.

How to Prevent It?

Know your ingredients. Read the notes on supply vendors' websites. If you have a fragrance oil that you know is going to accelerate, keep that batch simple. Keep temperatures in the 85°F to 90°F (29°C to 32°C) range. Don't discount the water too much. Oftentimes, mixing the fragrance oil in a few ounces (ml) of the warm soap oils first, before adding it to the rest of the soap, can help it perform better.

Soap that gets very hot/overheats in the mold may
- Crack down the middle during gel phase
- "Volcano" over the edges of the mold
- Contract on the top, looking like an "alien brain"
- Develop air tunnels through the center

These are all symptoms of a soap overheating in the mold. Many ingredients will cause a soap batch to heat up—milk, honey, sugars, juices, spice, and essential oils. If you include these in your soap, be aware. Keep your mixing temperatures on the low side (90°F to 100°F or 32°C to 38°C) and don't insulate the mold too heavily.

Two Problems Every Soap Maker Encounters Now and Then: DOS and Ash

Dreaded Orange Spots (DOS)

Most soap makers, at one time or another, encounter dreaded orange spots or DOS. These small orange spots are caused by oxidation of the free oils remaining in the soap as the superfat. Literally, the oil that's left behind in the batch of soap goes rancid. Fortunately, it's just an aesthetic problem. The soap is still safe to use, although in extreme cases, the oils that have oxidized/gone rancid may smell bad, too.

To prevent DOS:

- Keep your superfat levels under 10 percent, and keep the percentage of soft or fragile oils with short shelf lives (such as canola, rice bran, or sunflower) low.
- Make sure the oils and other ingredients you use are as fresh as possible. If you are going to keep oils on hand for a while, add an antioxidant such as vitamin E or rosemary oleoresin to the bottle.
- There is also some belief that using tap rather than distilled water can contribute to DOS.

Ash

Ash, or soda ash as is it sometimes called, is caused when free lye molecules that haven't combined with an oil molecule in the soap yet react with carbon dioxide in the air to make sodium carbonate. It is a white powdery substance that sticks to the surface of the soap, especially where the soap may have been exposed to the air as it was saponifying. It isn't harmful, other than looking bad.

Methods to combat ash:

- Spray the parts of your soap exposed to the air with rubbing alcohol about 15 minutes after you've poured the soap. I do this with all my batches.
- Cover the soap with plastic wrap to minimize contact with the air.
- Wait to unmold your soap until at least 36 to 48 hours after you pour the soap. Unmolding too soon seems to contribute to ash.

Methods to get rid of ash:

- Wipe it off with a moist cloth or buff it off with a nylon stocking.
- Steam it off using a handheld steamer.

Hot Process
Soap Making

Apart from two specialty soap recipes (see pages 157–163) that will be covered later in this section, hot process soap is not really a different method from cold process but, rather, *it is an added step*. The chemical reaction of the lye and the oils is the same—the difference is the added heat. It takes about 24 hours for the saponification process to complete in cold process soap and it also needs to cure for several weeks. Adding heat to the soap and, in effect, cooking it, hurries the saponification process and reduces the time in the mold to just a few hours, and the cure time to just 1 to 2 weeks.

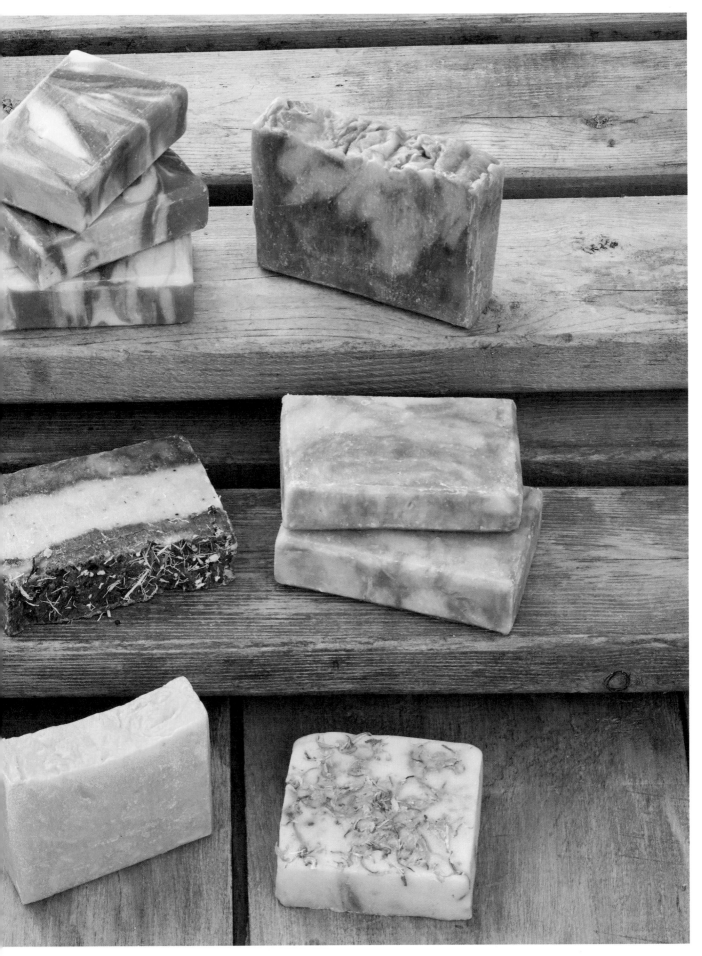

Why Hot Process?

The primary benefit of hot process soap making is the time saved. While the soap can benefit from additional cure time, it is essentially ready to use as soon as it comes out of the mold. Also, because additives are usually added after cooking, the hot process allows the use of additives that might otherwise cause problems, such as seizing in cold process batches or being diminished or scorched by the lye solution.

The primary disadvantage of hot process soap making is that the soap is not as fluid when poured into the mold and, hence, results in a thicker, more rustic look. But even this can be managed with careful preparation and a few simple techniques.

BASIC SLOW COOKER AND OVEN HOT PROCESS SOAP

There are two common methods to cooking the raw soap—in a slow cooker and in the oven. Both give comparable results and, depending on your slow cooker, take about the same amount of time. Slow cookers allow easier monitoring of the soap, but can heat unevenly and need to be stirred more often. Pots in the oven are more difficult to check, but heat much more evenly.

Start with a soap recipe that will make 3 pounds (1.36 kg) of soap. Use any soap recipe you like, but adjust it so the water amount is 2.5 times the lye amount. For example, the Basic recipe (page 86) calls for water equal to 2 times the amount of lye. For a standard 3-pound (1.36 kg) cold process batch of soap this would be 4.5 ounces (132 g) lye and 9 ounces (264 g) water. For hot process, multiply the lye by 2.5 times—or in this case, 11.25 ounces (319 g) water.

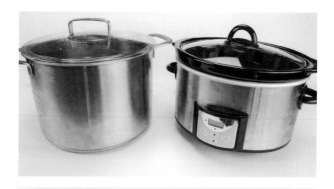

INGREDIENTS
- 1.5 tablespoons (22.5 g) plain yogurt
- 1.5 ounces (42.5 g) fragrance oil or essential oil

EQUIPMENT
- Slow cooker or oven
- Soap mold

Makes 3 pounds (1.36 kg)

1 Remove 20 percent of the total water needed for your recipe and set it aside. Make the lye solution with the remaining water.

2 Measure and melt the oils. Because you're adding heat to it, the temperatures at which you combine the lye and oils are not important, but should be under 170°F (77°C).

3 Mix the oils and lye to trace in the pot or slow cooker. Set the slow cooker on low or put the pot into a preheated 170°F to 180°F (77°C to 82°C) oven (A).

4 Place a piece of plastic wrap over the top of the pot and place the lid on the pot (B). This key step helps minimize the water lost during the cooking process.

5 After 20 minutes, lift the lid to check the soap. If you remove the plastic wrap, do so only for a moment. If it looks fluffier and more translucent around the edge of the pot, that is perfect (C).

6 Replace the lid and let it cook some more. If it has fluffed up to more than twice its original volume, the heat may be too high. Remove the plastic and stir the soap batter.

7 After another 20 minutes, check the soap again. It should, again, be fluffier and translucent, but reaching almost to the middle of the pot. Quickly remove the plastic and stir the soap. Replace the plastic and lid and let it continue to cook (D).

8 After about 20 minutes more, the soap should be fully cooked. It should look like a combination of petroleum jelly and applesauce. Remove it from the oven, or turn the slow cooker off (E).

9 Stir in the water held back from the lye solution, the yogurt, and add the fragrance or essential oils.

10 Add any additional colorants or additives and ladle the soap into your mold (F).

Note: As with all hot process soaps, this soap is ready to use as soon as it cools, but will benefit from a 1- to 2-week cure time.

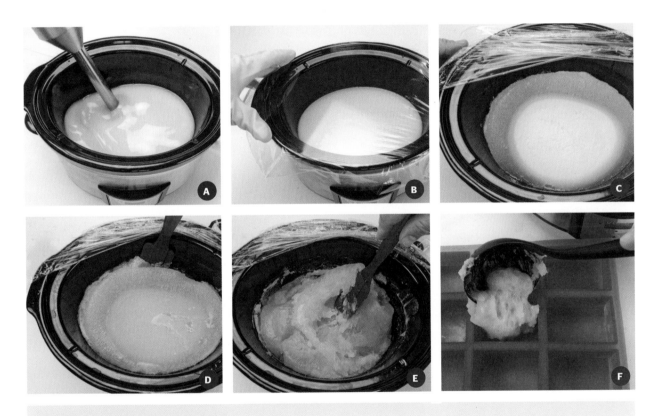

Sodium Lactate: Double Duty

Sodium lactate is often used in cold process soap recipes to make the soap harden more quickly. It does this as well for hot process soap, but it also helps the cooked soap batter remain more fluid in the pot. Use 1 teaspoon for every 1 pound (454 g) of oils.

You can also use 1 tablespoon (15 g) plain yogurt per 1 pound (454 g) of oils to make hot process soap much more stirrable and pourable.

Swirling Hot Process Soap

When it is done cooking, hot process soap is much thicker than cold process soap when it's first mixed. The soap thickens further as it is cools, making separating it into containers, adding colors, scooping it into the mold, and trying to get a swirl all quite a challenge. Here are two techniques that make swirling hot process soap easier. Both involve keeping the soap hot for as long as possible, holding back some water, and adding yogurt.

HOT PROCESS IN-THE-POT SWIRL

For this, use a soap recipe that will make 3 pounds (1.36 kg) of soap, with the water amount adjusted to 2.5 times the lye amount and 20 percent of the water set aside to add after cooking.

INGREDIENTS
- ½ teaspoon each of 4 mica colors
- 2 tablespoons (30 g) plain yogurt
- 1.5 ounces (42.5 g) fragrance oil or essential oil

EQUIPMENT
- 4 large measuring cups
- Chopstick or spatula

3 pounds (1.36 kg)

1 Mix the lye and heated oils.

2 Cook the soap using the slow cooker or oven method (see page 146). When the soap has finished cooking, stir it so it is evenly mixed.

3 Stir in the fragrance.

4 In each of the four containers, mix:
- One-fourth of the reserved water, heated
- ½ teaspoon mica
- 1.5 teaspoons yogurt (A)

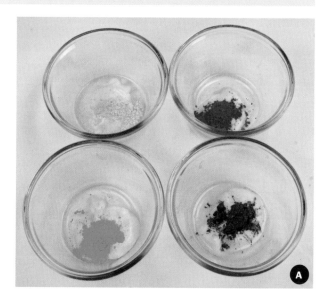

Mica and yogurt ready to be mixed

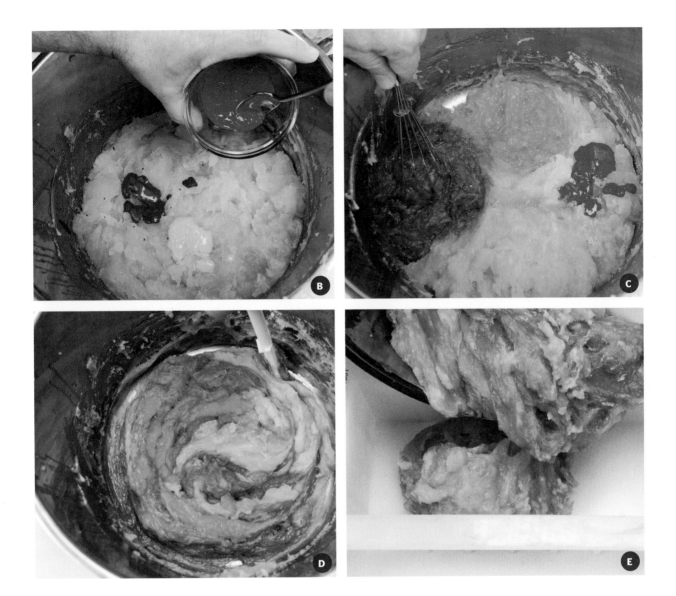

5 Pour the four colorant mixtures into the top, bottom, left, and right of the soap pot (B).

6 Whisk the colorant mixture into just that quadrant of soap (C).

7 Once you've mixed the colorant into all four quadrants of soap, use a chopstick or spatula to stir the soap in a spiral pattern, swirling as much as desired (D).

8 Pour or scoop the soap into the mold (E).

HOT PROCESS IN-THE-MOLD SWIRL

For these recipes, use a soap recipe that will make 3 pounds (1.36 kg) of soap, with the water amount adjusted to 2.5 times the lye amount and 20 percent of the water set aside to add after cooking.

INGREDIENTS

- ½ teaspoon each of 4 mica colors
- 1 teaspoon titanium dioxide
- 3 tablespoons (45 g) plain yogurt
- 1.5 ounces (44 ml) fragrance oil or essential oil

EQUIPMENT

- 4 medium-size (16 ounces or 454 g) glass containers
- 5 ramekins
- Medium-size container for mixing the reserved water and yogurt
- Soap mold
- Small spatula

Makes 3 pounds (1.36 kg)

1 Set aside 10 tablespoons (150 ml) of the soap oils.

2 Mix the lye and heated oils.

3 Cook the soap using the slow cooker or oven method (see page 146).

4 While the soap cooks, heat the glass containers in a 180°F (82°C) oven, along with any whisks, ramekins, and other soap tools you're using.

5 When the soap has finished cooking, stir it so it is evenly mixed.

6 Add the fragrance. Keep the soap heated until the colorants and additives are prepared.

7 Heat the 10 tablespoons (150 ml) reserved oils to 160°F (71°C) or so.

8 In each of four heated ramekins, mix

- ½ teaspoon mica
- 2 tablespoons (30 ml) warmed oils

9 To the remaining ramekin, add 2 tablespoons (30 ml) heated oils and the titanium dioxide.

10 In a separate container, mix the reserved water and yogurt and heat to 180°F (82°C).

11 Remove the cooked soap from the heat and stir in the water-yogurt mixture (A). Let it sit for 3 to 4 minutes.

12 Separate about half the soap into the four heated glass containers and stir 1 mica-oil mixture into each container.

13 Stir the titanium dioxide into the remaining soap (B).

14 Pour the white soap into the mold (C).

15 Alternate pouring the four colored soaps in zigzag lines into the white soap (D).

16 Tap the soap firmly on the counter to settle and flatten it (E).

17 Using a small spatula, swirl the soap, keeping the spatula at an angle to push as much colored soap as possible down into the white soap.

18 Repeat the zigzag swirls, as desired (F). Because the soap is so thick, the batter will take more swirling than with cold process soap before it gets muddy. Tap the soap onto the counter again.

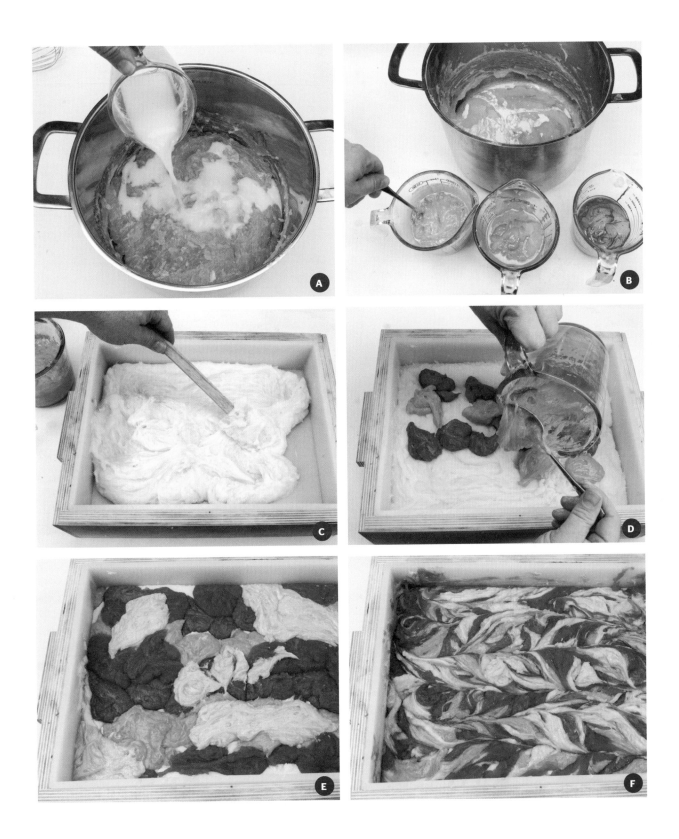

More Hot Process Soap Recipes

Although some soap makers use only hot process to make a batch quickly, others prefer the hot process method and take advantage of its differences. Here are some recipes that are particularly suited for hot process.

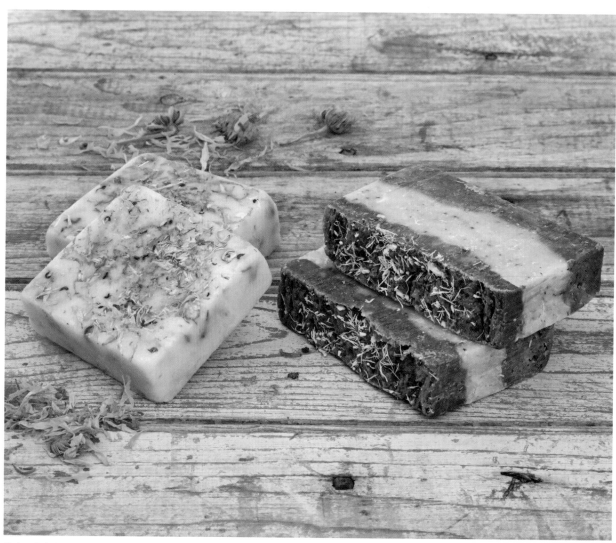

Calendula Hot Process Soap (left) and Layered Soap with Yucca Root (right).

LAYERED SOAP
WITH YUCCA ROOT

For this, use a recipe that will make 3 pounds (1.36 kg) of soap, with the water adjusted to 2.5 times the lye amount and 20 percent of the water set aside to add after cooking. This soap, shown opposite, right, embraces the rustic look of hot process soap by including a rustic-looking botanical—ground yucca root.

1 When the soap has finished cooking, stir in the fragrance oil, yogurt, and reserved water. Let it sit for 3 to 4 minutes.

2 Divide half the soap between the two containers. To one container, blend in the green mica (A); to the other, blend in the ground yucca root.

3 Scoop a layer of green soap into the mold, followed by the white/yucca soap layer (B).

4 Pour the remaining green soap onto the white layer.

5 Sprinkle some yucca root on top of the soap, pressing it gently so it will adhere (C).

INGREDIENTS

- 1.5 ounces (42.5 g) fragrance oil or essential oil
- 2 tablespoons (30 g) plain yogurt
- ½ teaspoon green mica
- 3 tablespoons (15 g) ground yucca root, plus more for sprinkling the soap

EQUIPMENT

- 2 large measuring cups
- Soap mold

Makes 3 pounds (1.36 kg)

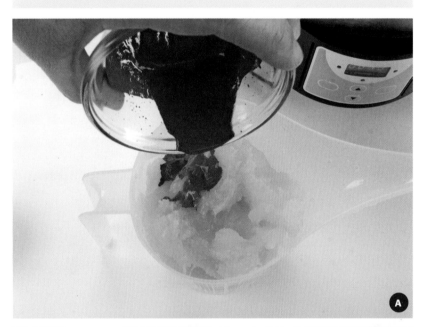

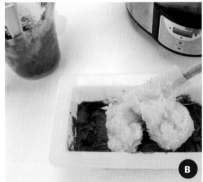

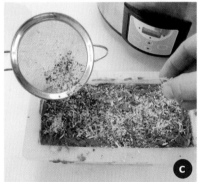

CALENDULA HOT PROCESS SOAP

For this, use a soap recipe that will make 3 pounds (1.36 kg) of soap, with the water adjusted to 2.5 times the lye amount and 20 percent of the water set aside to add after cooking.

1 Mix the lye and oils.

2 Cook the soap using the slow cooker or oven method (see pages 26–28). When the soap has finished cooking, stir it so it is evenly mixed.

3 Add the fragrance oil.

4 In a container, mix together the yogurt and reserved water. Heat to 180°F (82°C). Stir it into the cooked soap and let it sit for 3 to 4 minutes.

5 Sprinkle some calendula petals into the mold cavities (A).

6 Scoop the soap into the mold, being careful not to disturb the petals. The finished soap is shown on page 152, at left.

INGREDIENTS

- 1.5 ounces (42.5 g) fragrance oil or essential oil
- 2 tablespoons (30 g) plain yogurt
- 4 tablespoons (16 g) calendula petals

EQUIPMENT

- Container for mixing the yogurt and reserved water

Makes 3 pounds (1.36 kg)

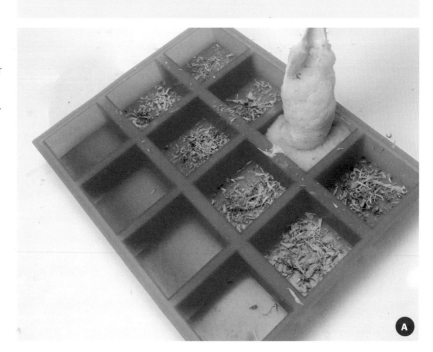

CARROT SOAP WITH SHREDS

For this soap, shown opposite, at left, start with a soap recipe that makes 3 pounds (1.36 kg) of soap, with the water adjusted to 2.5 times the lye amount, and 20 percent of the water set aside to add after cooking.

INGREDIENTS

- 1 lb (454 g) shredded soap
- ½ teaspoon orange mica
- 2 tablespoons (30 g) plain yogurt
- 3 ounces (85 g) carrot purée (see Note)
- 1.5 ounces (42.5 g) fragrance oil or essential oil

EQUIPMENT

- See Hot Process in-the-Pot Swirl (page 148)

Makes 3 pounds (1.36 kg)

1 Follow the instructions for the Hot Process in-the-Pot Swirl (page 148).

2 Sprinkle the orange mica onto the soap shreds and toss lightly to coat.

3 After cooking the soap, stir in the water–yogurt mixture, carrot purée, and fragrance. Let it sit for 3 to 4 minutes.

4 Stir the orange shreds into the cooked soap and scoop the soap into the mold.

Note: Cook 3 ounces (85 g) baby carrots in water until soft. Purée the carrots with 1 to 2 ounces (28 to 57 g) of water until smooth.

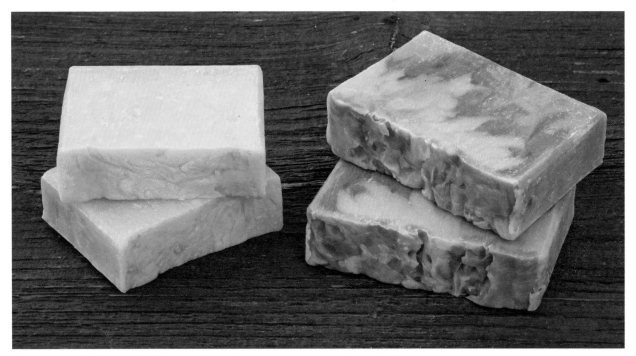

Carrot Soap with Shreds (left), Layered Lavender, Lemon, and Lime Soap (right).

LAYERED LAVENDER, LEMON, AND LIME SOAP

For this, shown above, use a recipe that makes 3 pounds (1.36 kg) of soap, with the water adjusted to 2.5 times the lye amount and 20 percent of the water set aside to add after cooking.

INGREDIENTS

- 2 tablespoons (30 g) plain yogurt
- ½ teaspoon green mica
- ½ teaspoon yellow mica
- ¼ teaspoon each blue and purple micas, mixed together
- 0.5 ounce (14 g) lavender essential oil
- 0.5 ounce (14 g) lemon essential oil
- 0.5 ounce (14 g) lime essential oil

EQUIPMENT

- See Hot Process in-the-Mold Swirl (page 150)
- Hanger swirl tool

Makes 3 pounds (1.36 kg)

1 Follow the instructions for the Hot Process In-the-Mold Swirl (page 150), including keeping all the containers and additives hot.

2 After cooking the soap and mixing in the water–yogurt mixture, divide the soap among three heated containers. Stir one mica–oil mixture into each container.

3 Pour the first soap color into the mold. Tap the mold firmly on the counter to settle the soap.

4 Pour the two remaining layers, firmly tapping again between layers.

5 Using a hanger swirl tool, swirl the soap as much as desired.

Specialty Hot Process Soap Recipes: Liquid and Cream Soaps

There are two special types of soap that work best using a hot process—liquid and cream soaps. Whereas sodium hydroxide is used to make hard bar soaps, these soaps utilize *potassium hydroxide* as (at least some of) the saponifying agent to make a liquid or creamy soap.

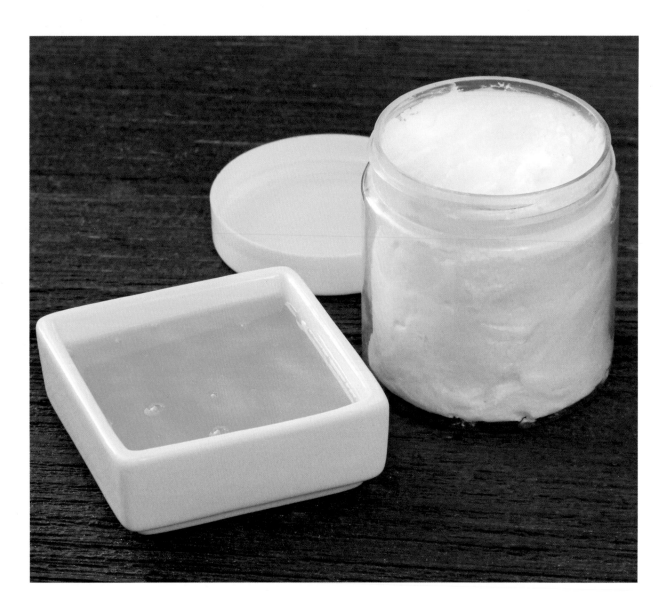

Formulating a Liquid Soap Recipe

As with any soap recipe, you can choose which oils you want to include, and these oils impart their qualities to the soap. Consider

- **Coconut oil:** As with bar soaps, it makes a great lathering soap. In liquid soap, it dissolves easily making for a very clear soap, but one that doesn't have a lot of thickness or body.
- **Liquid oils:** Oils such as olive, almond, and sunflower make a soap that doesn't lather as well, but is very easy to thicken with a saltwater solution.

- **Castor oil:** Castor oil is a very popular oil because it not only makes a very clear soap, but also can be thickened with saltwater.
- **Hard oils:** Oils such as palm oil, cocoa butter, and tallow can be used in liquid soap as well, however, the stearic acid in them makes a somewhat opaque soap. They can be thickened some with saltwater as well.

Which Oils to Choose

Liquid soap can be made from any of these oils. The balance that needs to be considered is primarily thickness versus lather. If you want a soap that will give abundant lather, but don't mind it being light and watery (or if you're going to use it in foaming containers), make a soap high in coconut oil. If you want a soap that more closely mimics the viscosity of commercial liquid soaps, formulate it primarily with liquid oils.

BUBBLY BUT THIN SOAP

INGREDIENTS
- 70 percent coconut oil
- 15 percent sunflower oil
- 15 percent castor oil

MILD BUT THICK SOAP

INGREDIENTS
- 50 percent olive oil
- 30 percent sunflower oil
- 20 percent castor oil

How to Make Liquid Soap

There are several phases to making liquid soap:

1 Make the soap paste

2 Dilute the paste

3 Neutralize/buffer the soap

4 Add fragrance or color

5 Thicken the soap

INGREDIENTS

- 4 ounces (113 g) potassium hydroxide
- 12 ounces (355 ml) water, plus 50 to 100 ounces (3 L) more for dilution
- 10 ounces (283.5 g) olive oil
- 6 ounces (170 g) sunflower oil
- 4 ounces (113 g) castor oil
- 1 ounce (28 g) borax
- 2 ounces (56.5) salt

EQUIPMENT

- Slow cooker or oven, for cooking the soap paste
- Whisk

Makes 48 ounces (1.36 kg) finished soap paste

1 Gather all your soap-making tools and weigh all your ingredients.

2 Using all safety precautions and wearing gloves and goggles, slowly add the potassium hydroxide to the water. Potassium hydroxide reacts more vigorously than sodium hydroxide and it will sound like it is boiling in the bottom of the pitcher. Just keep stirring until it is fully dissolved and set it aside in a safe place to cool to less than 180°F (82°C).

3 Heat the oils to between 150°F and 160°F (65.5°C and 71°C) and put them into the slow cooker (A).

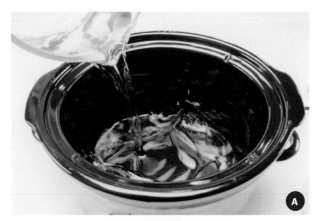

4 Slowly pour the lye solution into the heated oils while gently stirring with a whisk.

5 With the slow cooker set on low or the oven preheated to 180°F (82°C), begin blending with an immersion blender. The soap will thicken like bar soap, which will look like trace—but keep blending. As you blend, the soap batter will thicken and release several times, often looking like mashed potatoes or thick applesauce before it thickens (B). Keep blending. Recipes with a high percentage of liquid oils (like this one) may take 30 to 40 minutes to finally reach trace.

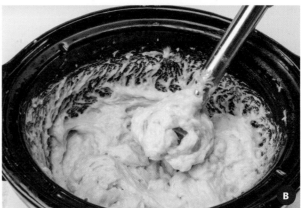

6 The soap will finally thicken to an opaque melted taffy-like consistency. It will be difficult to stir or even blend any more (C). This is the trace stage for liquid soap. Cover the pot and let it cook.

7 After 15 to 20 minutes, stir the soap to see if there is any separation. If so, stir it well and let it cook some more.

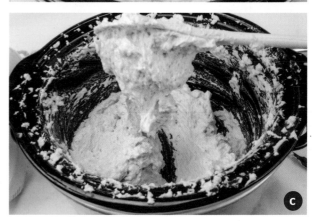

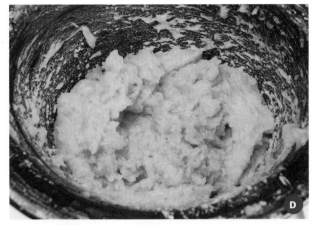

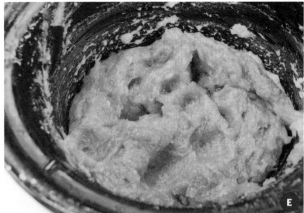

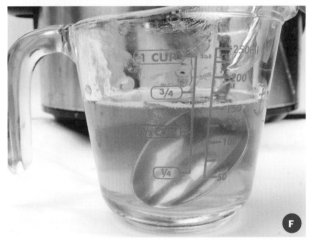

9 Cover the soap and let it cook, stirring every 30 to 45 minutes. The soap batter will begin to transform into a golden translucent paste and, over 2 to 3 hours, will become fully translucent (E).

10 Once the soap has finished cooking, test it for doneness by gently mixing 1 ounce (28 g) soap paste with 2 ounces (59 ml) g) boiling water. Let the mixture cool. If the diluted soap is clear, or just slightly cloudy, it is done cooking. If the soap appears milky or if there is a film floating on top, cook the paste for 1 hour more and do the test again.

11 The additional cooking time should finish cooking the paste. Give it another doneness test (see step 10). If it tests clear or just slightly cloudy, turn off the cooker and let the paste cool (F). If it is still milky, you may have measured too much oil into the recipe. The soap paste will still be useable, it will just be cloudy when diluted.

8 After another 15 to 20 minutes, check the soap again for separation and stir if necessary (D).

How Much Paste to Use and How Much Water to Add?

The preceding recipe, made entirely with liquid oils, makes 48 ounces (1.36 kg) of paste and requires about 72 ounces (2 L) of water to dilute fully. That's more than 7 pounds (3.2 kg) of finished soap. The paste will keep, refrigerated, for a long time, so only dilute as much paste as you need to make the soap you want. As a starting point, take 6 ounces (170 g) soap paste and dilute it with about 10 ounces (296 ml) water to make 1 pound (454 g) finished liquid soap.

DILUTE THE SOAP PASTE

There is one key requirement to diluting liquid soap paste—patience. The process is simple.

1 Measure the amount of soap paste you want to dilute (A).

2 Add enough (see page 159) hot water to the soap paste and gently stir enough to break up the soap chunks but not so much as to make too many bubbles (B).

3 If, after sitting for several hours, it congeals or forms a skin on the top of the pot, add a bit more hot water. Stir and let it sit for a few more hours. If it stays fluid, it's done (C)!

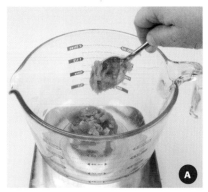
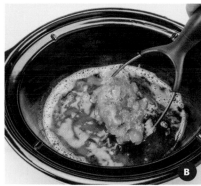
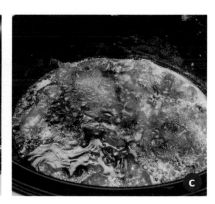

NEUTRALIZING AND BUFFERING THE SOAP PASTE

As with bar soap, superfatting your recipe—as it's supposed to—leaves a bit of unsaponified oil in the finished soap. In liquid soap, however, this results in cloudy soap. So, liquid soap recipes are generally formulated with 0 percent superfat. To buffer any excess lye, the soap is neutralized using a borax solution.

1 Mix 1 ounce (28 g) borax with 4 ounces (113 g) very hot water.

2 Add 2 tablespoons (15 ml) borax solution for every 1 pound (454 g) of *undiluted* soap paste.

For example, if you use 8 ounces (226.8 g) soap paste and add 12 ounces (340 g) water to dilute it, you would add 1 tablespoon (15 ml) borax solution (again, based on the weight of the *undiluted* soap paste) to neutralize and buffer it.

ADD FRAGRANCE OR COLOR

Some fragrance oils can affect liquid soap in strange ways, causing them to thicken, break down, or turn cloudy. Stir ½ teaspoon fragrance oil into 3 ounces (85 g) warmed soap. Let it sit for 30 minutes to see what effect it may have. If it tests fine, add 0.2 to 0.3 ounce (5.6 to 8.5 g), or 1 to 2 percent, for every 1 pound (454 g) of soap.

THICKEN THE SOAP PASTE

There are two easy options for giving your soap more thickness—additional borax or saltwater. Borax works best with coconut oil. Saltwater works wonderfully with liquid oils. For recipes with some of both type of oils, you can try a bit of both.

To use borax:

1 Heat the diluted soap and borax solution used to about 150°F (65.5°C) to neutralize it.

2 Add 1 tablespoon (15 ml) borax solution per 1 pound (454 g) of **diluted** soap.

3 Let the soap cool to room temperature. Test the thickness. If you want a thicker soap, add 1 additional tablespoon (15 ml) borax solution.

To use saltwater:

4 Fully dissolve 1 ounce (28 g) salt in 4 ounces (113 g) hot water.

5 To room temperature soap, start with ½ teaspoon saltwater solution per 1 pound (454 g) of diluted soap. Stir well and let the soap sit for at least 1 hour.

6 Repeat to increase the thickness of the soap. Recipes made with liquid oils can be thickened to an almost gel-like consistency using a saltwater solution!

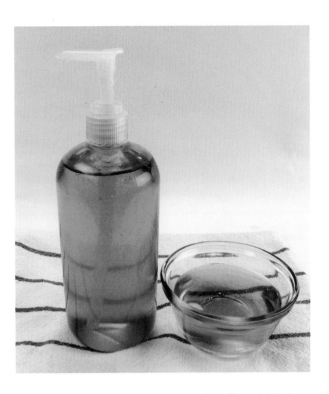

Once the soap is diluted, many soap makers like to let it sit for 1 to 2 weeks to settle. Often, any impurities that made the soap slightly cloudy will settle out. If this happens, gently pour the clear soap into another bottle and discard the small amount of settled particles in the bottom of the jar.

Cream Soap

Cream soap is a hot process soap that uses both sodium hydroxide and potassium hydroxide to make a soap that is firm, but scoopable—a bit thicker and heavier than whipped cream. It is wonderful as a body wash or shaving soap.

BASIC CREAM SOAP

INGREDIENTS

- 3.2 ounces (91 g) potassium hydroxide
- 0.7 ounce (20 g) sodium hydroxide
- 22 ounces (623.7 g) water
- 10 ounces (283.5 g) stearic acid
- 4.5 ounces (127.5 g) coconut oil
- 3 ounces (85 g) sunflower oil
- 1.5 ounces (42.5 g) castor oil
- 5.5 ounces (156 g) glycerin
- 0.5 ounce (14 g) boric acid dissolved in 4 ounces (113 g) hot water
- 1 to 1.5 ounces (28 to 42.5 g) fragrance oil or essential oil

EQUIPMENT

- Various containers for melting and combining ingredients
- Slow cooker
- Immersion blender

Makes 3 pounds (1.36 kg) cream soap

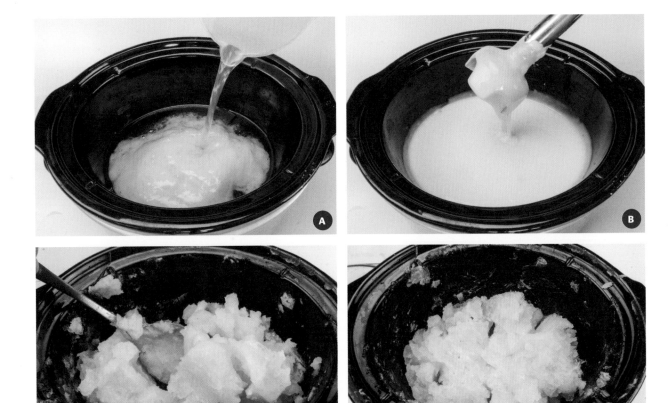

1. Add the sodium and potassium hydroxide to the water. Stir and set aside.

2. Melt the stearic acid by itself.

3. Into the melted stearic acid, melt the coconut oil.

4. Add the liquid oils.

5. Pour the oils into a slow cooker set on high heat.

6. Add the lye to the oils and blend with the immersion blender (A).

7. As with liquid soap, it will go through several stages where it looks like:

   - Liquid melted milkshake (B)
   - Watery/lumpy mashed potatoes
   - Creamy honey

8. Once the soap reaches the honey stage, give it one more stir, cover the cooker, and let the soap cook.

9. Check the soap every 30 minutes, stirring if the soap begins to rise. The soap will likely get very thick after an hour or so, so you'll more be chunking and turning it in the pot rather than stirring (C).

10. After 3 to 4 hours of cooking time, the soap should be uniformly golden and translucent. Turn the heat off and let it sit in the pot for 24 hours (D).

(continued)

(continued)

11 Transfer the soap to a large bowl and add the boric acid solution (E).

12 Using your immersion blender, blend the soap. Quite amazingly, the soap will suddenly begin to lighten and become lighter and fluffier (F).

13 Continue blending until the soap is smooth and fluffy (G). Whip in any color and fragrance oil desired and let the soap rest for several hours.

14 If, after sitting, the soap is firmer than you like, add a bit more water, 1 tablespoon (15 ml) at a time until it is creamier. If it is not firm enough, add an additional 0.25 ounce (7 g) of boric acid dissolved in 1 ounce (30 ml) of water.

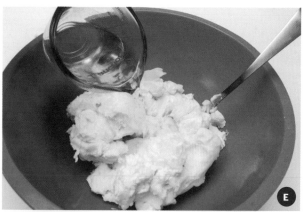

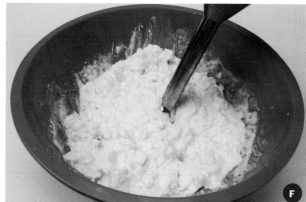

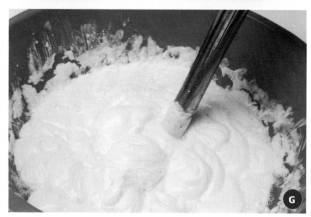

Hot Process Soap Making: Tips and Troubleshooting

All of the tips and solutions for cold process soap making also apply to hot process. It's important to measure accurately, mix well, and understand your ingredients. With hot process, however, there are two additional things to watch—heat and liquid.

Tips for Hot Process Soap Making

1 Prewarm as many of your utensils and ingredients as possible.
   - Warm your measuring cups, utensils, and ramekins in the oven
   - Mix your colorants with hot water or oil
   - Warm any milk or yogurt you are adding to the batch

2 Be sure to use enough liquid in the lye solution. Instead of the water being 2 times the weight of the lye, 2.5 times will give you more fluid soap.

3 The addition of milk, yogurt, and/or sodium lactate makes the soap much more fluid.

4 Use plastic wrap over the top of the pot to help retain moisture.

5 Stir sparingly. Each time you take the lid and plastic off of the pot, you lose heat and moisture.

6 Keep the temperature between 150°F to 170°F (66°C to 77°C). Slow and steady is the best way to cook hot process soap.

7 Embrace the thicker, more rustic look of hot process by designing your recipes with that in mind.

Troubleshooting

1 Soap with lumps and/or lighter-colored bits of soap mixed into the rest of the batch:
   - As the soap cooks, it will get dryer and lighter in color, but if the soap heats unevenly, the edges of the batch may cook more quickly than the center. Scraping the outer edge of the batch and stirring it back into the center as it is cooking will help minimize this.

2 Soap that is too thick to swirl or mold:
   - See the tips above. Using enough liquid and using additives are the best way to keep your soap more fluid.

3 Soap that separates in the pot:
   - Like cold process soap separating in the mold, this is a mixing problem, but one that is easy to fix. Just restir the soap well and let it continue to cook.

4 Soap with missing or light fragrance:
   - Some fragrance or essential oils (especially those with citrus constituents) can flash off (evaporate) from the heat in the soap. Use scent oils or blends with flash points greater than 150°F (66°C) to minimize this.

Mixing It Up—Further Soap-Making Adventures

Once you have several batches of soap under your belt, and have tried a couple of the various methods of soap making outlined in this book, you'll probably want to start experimenting. Great! Experimenting with different ingredients, techniques, and processes will help you learn more and enjoy making soap even more. Here are some suggestions for experimentation.

Mix Up Your Ingredients

After you have tried some batches with special ingredients like salt, milk, alternate liquids, or other additives try using more than one at a time. For example:

- Combine goat's milk (see page 105) with a soleseife/salt soap (see page 116) for super dense, creamy lather.

- Make a beer soap (see page 108) with added honey (see page 84) and the natural colorant of your choice.

- Make a batch splitting the lye solution made half with an alternate liquid and half with plain water. Mix the half batches separately, then swirl them together.

Mix Up Your Oils

Learn more about how different oils affect the qualities of your soap by experimenting with different oils and combinations. Be sure to keep all of the other conditions (temperature, liquids, etc.) the same, and take notes on the batch from start to finish including how long it takes to come to trace.

- Start by substituting just one of the oils in the recipe, keeping all of the other aspects of the recipe (e.g., water to lye ratio, temperature, fragrances) the same. Start with substituting an oil in the same category as the original. (e.g., substituting lard or tallow for palm oil or substituting almond oil for sunflower oil)

- Next, change the overall balance of the recipe (e.g., change the olive oil percentage from 30 to 50 percent and leaving the other oils in approximately the same proportion.

ORIGINAL RECIPE	ADJUSTED RECIPE
30% olive oil →	50% olive oil
25% palm oil →	18% palm oil
25% coconut oil →	18% coconut oil
20% sunflower oil →	14% sunflower oil

ORIGINAL RECIPE	ADJUSTED RECIPE
30% olive oil	30% olive oil
25% palm oil	25% palm oil
25% coconut oil	25% coconut oil
20% sunflower oil →	20% soybean oil

Mix Up Your Techniques

Ultimately, soap is soap no matter what technique you use to make it, but don't be limited to just one. Combine different methods for unique hybrid soaps. The results are limited only by your imagination and willingness to experiment.

1   Add premade, hand-milled shreds into a batch of melt and pour, cold or hot process soap. Each combination will give a different effect.

2   Add chunks of colored, clear melt and pour soap to a cold process batch. The mix of transparent and opaque can be wonderful.

3   Create a layered soap with layers of melt and pour and cold process soap.

4   Swirl melted melt and pour soap into a batch of cold, hot, or rebatched soap.

Mix Up Your Own Scent Blends

As I discussed earlier, the scents are one of the most pleasurable aspects of soap making, and creating your own scent blends can be one of the most gratifying. Scent blending (with either fragrance or essential oils) can be as simple as just mixing two together (e.g., vanilla and mint, lavender and orange). There are two simple blending techniques that I like to use; blending categories (see page 21) and blending notes.

Blending categories (e.g., woodsy, floral, citrus) works well with fragrance oils that are already blends of various scent constituents, natural and synthetic. Even a simple fragrance oil called lavender can be a mix of many ingredients as well as individual essential oils.

Blending notes works well with essential oils as they are more unique in their characteristics. Scent notes work very much like musical notes with (high) top, middle and (low) base notes.

Top note oils are light, bright, crisp, and full of energy. They generally have a fresh, immediately apparent quality that is intense, but fleeting, due to their fast evaporation rate. Examples of top note oils are bergamot, eucalyptus, grapefruit, lemon, mints, and pine.

Middle note oils are strong, lasting and potent without being overpowering. They may not be as bright and energetic as top notes but are, instead, bold and sturdy. Their scent emerges shortly after the top note's first impression. Examples of middle note oils are cinnamon, clove, geranium, juniper, lavender, rosemary, and tea tree.

Base note oils are the slowest to evaporate. Their rich, heavy scents emerge slowly and linger. They form the base of the fragrance and give it staying power. Examples of base note oils are benzoin, cedarwood, clove, patchouli, sandalwood, and vanilla.

Creating Your Own Scents

I have two basic rules for creating essential oil blends:

Rule 1: Create your blend with a balance of top, middle, and base notes (30%/50%/20% is a good starting point), and with the scent categories in mind.

Rule 2: Ignore rule 1 and just create blends with scents that you like. Experiment. Don't be afraid to create a blend of entirely "top notes." Even by themselves, essential oils are very complex, and these categories are generalizations. Many essential oils can contribute multiple "notes" to a blend or will act differently in relationship to others. For example, anise essential oil acts like a top note when blended with cinnamon and lavender, but more of a middle note when blended with a citrus oil like lemon or lime.

SUGGESTIONS FOR BUILDING YOUR ESSENTIAL OIL CABINET	
1 Lavender 40/42 – My "desert island" oil. I use it in most all of the blends I make. A little bit floral and a little bit herbaceous, it's versatile and blends well with practically everything.	**6 Cinnamon or clove –** Spicy notes – used in small quantities, they both add warmth and exoticness.
2 Rosemary – Wonderful in blends and gives a versatile, crisp, green complexity.	**7 Benzoin or balsam Peru –** Sweet, vanilla-like base notes. Gives a more warm, round note than patchouli or cedar wood.
3 Orange – Balances and rounds out blends making them cheery and sweet.	**8 Clary Sage –** A bittersweet floral with herbaceous and woodsy characteristics.
4 Patchouli or cedarwood – Earthy, woodsy, base notes —use them to anchor blends and give warmth and weight to your scent blends.	**9 Lemon –** Crisper and brighter than orange with the same citrus energy.
5 Mints – Spearmint and peppermint blend well with other essential oils. Spearmint is gentler and sweeter. Peppermint is bold and crisp. Use both sparingly.	**10 Geranium –** A definite floral note. Blends well with many other EOs.

Tips for fragrance and essential oil blending

Make sure to write everything down. If you find a blend you really like, you're going to want to duplicate it.

1   Make sure to give the blend time to mix and mature. In addition to smelling it when first mixed, store it in a sealed jar and smell it after several hours and after a couple of days.

2   As with substituting out just one oil in a soap recipe to see what effect it has on the final soap, substitute out just one oil in the essential oil blend to see what effect it has. For example, with a lavender, tea tree, and patchouli blend, try substituting rosemary for the tea tree or using half rosemary and half tea tree. You'll start to be able to discern the subtle differences of the oils and how they relate to the other essential oils.

3   Start a cabinet of essential oils to experiment with. Purchasing essential oils can be intimidating and expensive. Most of them will keep for several years if stored properly, so many soap makers will purchase essential oils one at a time, building their cabinet over time. Look for sales online or group purchases in one of the various soap-making communities.

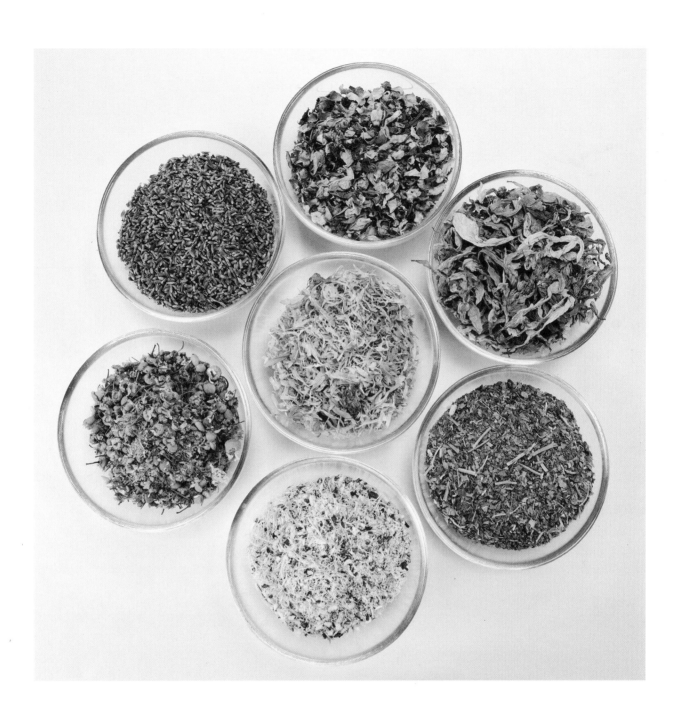

Resources

Supplies

There are dozens of great vendors of oils, fragrance and essential oils, colorants, packaging, equipment, and more. Those listed below are vendors from whom I have personally purchased supplies over the years.

Bramble Berry
www.brambleberry.com

Bulk Apothecary
www.bulkapothecary.com

Camden-Grey Essential Oils
www.camdengrey.com

Chemistry Store
www.chemistrystore.com

Columbus Foods
www.soaperschoice.com

Essential Depot
www.essentialdepot.com

From Nature with Love
www.fromnaturewithlove.com

Jedwards International
www.bulknaturaloils.com

Lebermuth Company
www.lebermuth.com

Liberty Natural
www.libertynatural.com

Mad Micas
www.madmicas.com

Majestic Mountain Sage
www.thesage.com

Nashville Wraps
www.nashvillewraps.com

New Directions Aromatics
www.newdirectionsaromatics.com

Nurture Soap
www.nurturesoap.com

Old Will Knot Scales
www.oldwillknotscales.com

Rustic Escentuals
www.rusticescentuals.com

San Francisco Herb Co.
www.sfherb.com

Shay and Company
www.shayandcompany.com

SKS Bottle and Packaging
www.sks.com

Soapalooza
www.soapalooza.com

Soap Equipment
www.soapequipment.com

Wellington Fragrance Company
www.wellingtonfragrance.com

Wholesale Supplies Plus
www.wholesalesuppliesplus.com

Communities

One of the best ways to get information, recommendations, ideas, and tips about soap-making is to join soap maker communities. You'll find kindred souls who love making soap as much as you do.

Handcrafted Soap and Cosmetics Guild
www.soapguild.org

Alabama Soap and Candle Assoc.
www.alabamasoapmeeting.com

Business of Soap Making
www.facebook.com/groups/modern-soapmakingmastermind

Canadian Guild of Soapmakers, Chandlers and Cosmetic Makers
www.canadianprofessionalsoapmakers.com

Florida Soap Crafters Gathering
http://floridasoapcrafters.blogspot.com

Handcrafted Bath & Body Guild of Canada
http://hbbg.ca

Indie Business Network
https://indiebusinessnetwork.com

I Saponify, No Lye
www.facebook.com/groups/isaponifynolye

Lone Star Soap and Toiletries
www.lonestarsoapandtoiletries.com

Lovin' Soap
www.lovinsoap.com

Make More Soap
www.makemoresoap.com

Modern Soapmaking
www.modernsoapmaking.com

Northeast Bubbles and Blazes
www.nebubblesandblazes.com

Ohio Soapers
http://ohiosoapers.blogspot.com

Saponification Nation
www.facebook.com/groups/saponificationnation

Soap Making Forum
www.soapmakingforum.com

Tennessee Soap and Candle
www.tnsoapandcandle.com

The Dish Forum
www.thedishforum.com/forum

If you have a supplier or community to recommend and add to the list, visit www.makemoresoap.com and let me know!

Acknowledgments

This book would not have been possible without the excitement, patience, flexibility, and support of my partner Robert and son Bennett, who have put up with months and months of soap-covered counters, tables, sinks, carts, and shelves. Additionally, thanks are due to Duncan for his encouragement and perserverance in the Bath Rabbit Soap Company and About.com years, for they allowed me to become the writer and soap maker that I am today. My gratitude and heartfelt appreciation go out to soap makers such as Kathy Miller, Sandy Maine, Maggie Hanus, Joyce Douglas, Michael Cook, Marie Gale, Donna Maria Coles Johnson, and Norma Coney, who freely shared their knowledge and inspired me in the beginning years (and still!), and the soap-making rock stars of today such as Anne-Marie Faiola, Kenna Cote, Amanda and Benjamin Aaron, Marla Bosworth, Charlene Simon, Holly Port, Beth Byrne, Leigh O'Donnell, Clara Lindberg, Kevin Dunn, and so many more, who each brings a unique style and perspective to making soap, but, as I do, share an almost unexplainable universal love for it as well.

Sincere thanks are also due to Joy Aquilino and the creative team at Quarto. Their guidance and patience were vital and graciously given. This project was far bigger than I ever expected it to be—but, through it, my love and respect for the art and craft of soap making has been reignited.

About the Author

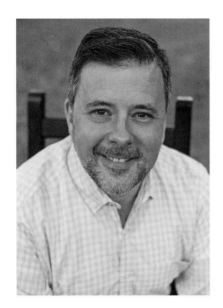

David Fisher has been exploring the art, science, and craft of making soap for nearly twenty years. His soap making quickly grew from a hobby into a small business—the Bath Rabbit Soap Company—and, in 2005, he transitioned from making and selling soap to making and *teaching* about soap. For eleven years, he was the guide to soap and candle making for About.com, writing hundreds of articles for an international audience, and is now writer and curator for MakeMore-Soap.com. David has been a teacher and speaker at numerous gatherings and conferences, including the Handcrafted Soap and Cosmetic Guild. When not making soap, he is the assistant director of cultural affairs for the City of Dallas, where he lives with his partner Robert and son Bennett.

Index